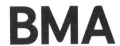

BMA Library

- Web access to all services
- Support helpdesk
- PDF articles to your mailbox
- Free online searches
- Wireless reading room
- Medline access

D1351417

By borrowing any item you are accepting the following conditio

1. The item must be returned to the BMA Library, please see ou details below.
2. The item is loaned until the date stamped, unless renewed.
3. Long-term loan items can be recalled after one month if required by another user.
4. **PROOF OF POSTAGE RECEIPT required from Post Office, if returning items by post, otherwise you will be liable for lost items.**

BMA Library, British Medical Association,
BMA House, Tavistock Square, London WC1H 9JP
Tel: 020 7383 6625

bma.org.uk/library

British Medical Association

We dedicate this book to the memory of Simon Newell, previous co-author of this book, and our friend and colleague.

Paediatrics
Lecture Notes

Jonathan C. Darling

MD MRCP FRCPCH FHEA MBChB
Clinical Associate Professor in Paediatrics and Child Health and Medical Education
Honorary Consultant Paediatrician
University of Leeds and Leeds Children's Hospital, Leeds Teaching Hospitals NHS Trust

James Yong

MRCPCH MBChB
Consultant Paediatrician and Honorary Senior Lecturer
Leeds Children's Hospital, Leeds Teaching Hospitals NHS Trust and University of Leeds

Tenth edition

WILEY Blackwell

This edition first published 2022

© 2022 John Wiley & Sons Ltd

Edition History

Previous editions published 1973, 1975, 1978, 1981, 1986, 1991, 2002, 2008 by Blackwell Publishing and 2014 by John Wiley & Sons Ltd.

Registered Offices

John Wiley & Sons, Inc., 111 River Street, Hoboken, NJ 07030, USA

John Wiley & Sons Ltd, The Atrium, Southern Gate, Chichester, West Sussex, PO19 8SQ, UK

Editorial Office

9600 Garsington Road, Oxford, OX4 2DQ, UK

For details of our global editorial offices, customer services, and more information about Wiley products visit us at www.wiley.com.

Wiley also publishes its books in a variety of electronic formats and by print-on-demand. Some content that appears in standard print versions of this book may not be available in other formats.

Library of Congress Cataloging-in-Publication Data

Names: Darling, Jonathan C., author. | Yong, James (Pediatrician), author.
  | Newell, Simon J. Lecture notes. Paediatrics.
Title: Lecture notes. Paediatrics / Jonathan C. Darling, James Yong.
Other titles: Paediatrics
Description: 10th edition. | Hoboken, NJ : Wiley-Blackwell, 2021. |
  Preceded by Lecture notes. Paediatrics / Simon J. Newell, Jonathan C.
  Darling. Ninth edition. 2014. | Includes bibliographical references and
  index.
Identifiers: LCCN 2020035532 (print) | LCCN 2020035533 (ebook) | ISBN
  9781119552871 (paperback) | ISBN 9781119552895 (adobe pdf) | ISBN
  9781119552918 (epub)
Subjects: MESH: Pediatrics-methods | Child Development-physiology
Classification: LCC RJ61 (print) | LCC RJ61 (ebook) | NLM WS 100 | DDC
  618.92–dc23
LC record available at https://lccn.loc.gov/2020035532
LC ebook record available at https://lccn.loc.gov/2020035533

Cover Design: Wiley
Cover Image: © sturti/Getty Images

Set in 8.5/11pt Utopia by Straive, Pondicherry, India

Printed in Singapore
M094441_290721

Contents

OSCE stations

Foreword

Fifty years ago when Dick Smithells and I were planning the first edition of *Lecture Notes on Paediatrics*, nearly all text books had a hard cover, and were large and expensive. Usually, the text was dense, diagrams and illustrations scanty and photographs (if present at all) confined to a few pages in the middle or end of the book. We wanted a less expensive book with a soft cover, which was small enough to fit in the pocket of the white coat worn (then) by medical students. We hoped to produce an attractive book by including many line drawings, charts and diagrams – unusual at that time. Unavoidably, everything had to be black and white, which was sadly inappropriate for the subject: children and families bring much colour to our lives.

We aimed for a book that

- 'describes the pattern of childhood growth and development and conditions that are either common, important or interesting. This factual framework is set against the changing pattern of paediatric practice, the services available to children and the needs of society'
- provides 'a framework of paediatric knowledge sufficient for the medical student during the paediatric appointment; but it must be grafted on to preliminary experience of adult medicine and surgery – with more emphasis on diagnosis than on treatment; therapeutic details are best learnt by caring for sick children'.

That 1973 first edition of Meadow and Smithells' *Lecture Notes* recorded the recent introduction of measles immunization, and the abandonment of smallpox vaccination. It still needed a lengthy section on congenital rubella and an even longer one on rhesus haemolytic disease of the newborn. Infant mortality was nearly five times greater than today, as was childhood death in the United Kingdom from infection. There was a succinct account of battered babies, recently defined, but no mention of other forms of child abuse – yet to be recognized and described.

After six editions, Smithells retired and was succeeded by Simon Newell our former student and trainee. His appointment made us happy, and his early death very, very sad. His spirit and his innovations (as well as some splendid drawings by his daughter, then a schoolgirl) live on in this 10th edition, now with Jonathan Darling, another former trainee, as the lead author.

The book still contains much of the original structure, text and illustrations from the first edition. But this new Darling and Yong edition is worthy of its time – up to date with an attractive colourful format, and increased use of illustrations, information boxes, teaching points and advice on preparing for clinical examinations. The authors and production team have produced the sort of book that Meadow and Smithells hoped for long ago. It is perhaps larger than they hoped for; but children grow, paediatrics advances and expands, and the students of today are capable and worthy.

Children make up one fifth of the population. Doctors dealing with them and their families are fortunate because paediatrics is worthwhile, fulfilling and fun. This book will help you to understand, wonder and better contribute to the future.

Roy Meadow 2021
Emeritus Professor of Paediatrics
and Child Health, University of Leeds
Lead author for the first seven editions
of Lecture Notes: Paediatrics

Preface

Paediatrics is a wonderful specialty of medicine! You might think us biased in saying that (we are), but we hope in your journey through paediatrics that you will discover something of the truth of that for yourself. In what other specialty can you be a true generalist or a tertiary specialist, work in the community or in intensive care, or deal with the care of extremely premature babies through to the challenges of adolescence?

And knowledge of paediatrics is relevant in many other career pathways, ranging from primary care to many surgical specialties and anaesthetics.

Children are 20% of the population and are seen in 40% of general practice consultations. We have again set out to focus on the core of the paediatric curriculum that every medical student should learn. We hope our book will also be useful to all other health professionals who care for children.

In the 10th edition, we have continued the use of information boxes indicating *key points, practice points, treatment guides, learning logs* and web-based support material. Each chapter begins with a chapter map and suggests practical ways of gaining experience in paediatrics in the learning log at the end.

Students and teachers all want success in examinations. To help you prepare, the OSCE stations, tips and self-test questions at the end of each chapter can be used alongside the section on *Preparing for Clinical Examinations in Paediatrics and Child Health* and the extended matching questions (EMQs).

The book has an easy-to-follow structure: Part 1 takes you through the essentials you need to know at the outset; Part 2 covers normal and abnormal from foetal life through to adolescence; then Part 3 moves to systems and specialties; and finally, we explain in Part 4 what happens next – exams and (we hope) careers in paediatrics.

We both used *Lecture Notes* as medical students, and it is a popular choice of text at home in the UK and abroad. We hope you will enjoy reading it during your paediatrics, and that it will in some way contribute to still higher and better standards for children's health during your careers in the next 40 years.

Jonathan C. Darling
James Yong

Acknowledgements

This book was conceived by Professor Sir Roy Meadow and Professor Dick Smithells, whose teaching inspired many students in paediatrics. Our colleague, Simon Newell then brought his expert and enthusiastic touch to the book over several editions. We continue to build on the foundation they laid – their voices can still be heard in these pages.

We are grateful to the European Resuscitation Council for permission to use their illustrations and algorithms in emergency paediatrics. We thank the focus groups of medical students, whose reflections on the previous edition were so helpful to us.

Further reading

Large comprehensive textbooks:

Kliegman, R.M., St Geme, J.W., Blum, N.J. et al. (eds.) (2019). Nelson Textbook of Pediatrics, 21e. Elsevier.

McIntosh, N., Helms, P.J., Smyth, R.L., and Logan, S. (eds.) (2008). Forfar and Arneil's Textbook of Pediatrics, 7e. Churchill Livingstone.

Zitelli, B.J., SC, M.I., and Nowalk, A.J. (2018). Atlas of Pediatric Physical Diagnosis, 7e. Elsevier.

Rennie, J.M. (ed.) (2012). Rennie & Roberton's Textbook of Neonatology, 5e. Churchill Livingstone.

Levene, M.I. and Tenore, A. (2011). European Mastercourse in Paediatrics (European Academy of Paediatrics and Royal College of Paediatrics and Child Health). Churchill Livingstone.

We have included links to useful supplementary reading and resources throughout the text – look out for the grey boxes.

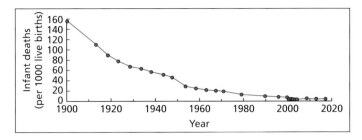

Figure 1.4 Infant mortality (0–1 years). By 2000, the infant mortality in England and Wales had fallen to a fraction of the level in 1900 (from 156 per 1000 live births to 5.6 per 1000). It has continued to fall further, to 3.8 in 2018. Even in the last 30 years it has fallen by nearly 60%.

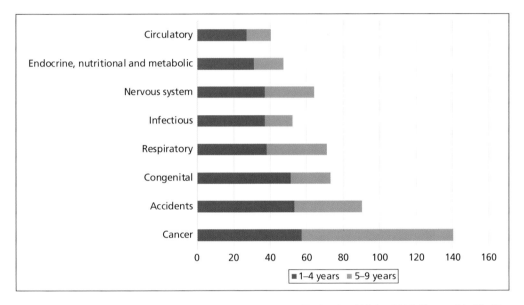

Figure 1.5 Leading causes of death in children aged 1 to 9 years. England and Wales 2018. *Source:* Modified from Office for National Statistics. https://stateofchildhealth.rcpch.ac.uk/evidence/mortality/child-mortality/.

1.3.3 Childhood morbidity

- The pattern of morbidity in children is very different from that of adults (Figure 1.6):
  - Infections are common, especially of the respiratory, gastrointestinal and urinary tracts, as well as the acute exanthemata (e.g. chickenpox).
  - Degenerative disorders and cerebral vascular accidents are very rare.
- New forms of chronic disease are becoming relatively more important as formerly fatal childhood disorders become treatable (but not necessarily curable):
  - Children with complex congenital heart disease, malignant disease, cystic fibrosis and renal failure benefit from modern life-saving therapies

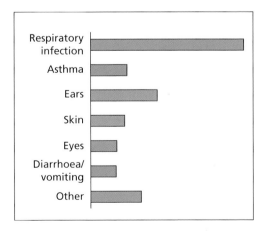

Figure 1.6 Most common reasons for a child to be seen by their GP.

but may not achieve a cure and often have to live with the difficulties and side effects of complicated treatment.

The hallmarks of childhood are growth and development, which influence both the kinds and the patterns of childhood illness. Congenital malformations, genetic disease and the consequences of problems in the perinatal period (e.g. cerebral palsy) are common. You do not need to spend much time looking after children to realize that disturbances of development and behaviour, and anxiety about normal variants, are both prevalent and important to parents.

It has been estimated that a British GP with an average practice would see a new case of pyloric stenosis every 4 years, childhood diabetes every 6 years, Down syndrome every 16 years, Turner syndrome every 60 years and haemophilia or Hirschsprung disease every 600 years! Hospitals may give a very false impression of the pattern of illness in the community at large.

1.4 Children in society

1.4.1 Socioeconomic inequalities

Socioeconomic status is a key determinant of child health. The health and educational progress of a child is directly related to the home and the environment. The infant mortality rate in the most deprived areas of England is nearly twice that of the least deprived (see Figure 1.7), and a similar pattern is seen in child mortality rates and most other population health indicators. The disadvantage is there at birth and continues throughout childhood. In many developed countries, health inequalities have grown wider even as average health levels have improved.

The UK has one of the worst rates of child poverty in the industrialized world. The proportion of UK

 RESOURCE

State of Child Health in the UK (**https://stateofchildhealth.rcpch.ac.uk**) summarizes key data.
The 'Child and Maternal Health' section of the Public Health England website (**https://fingertips.phe.org.uk**) enables you to explore and compare local data.

 RESOURCE

See **www.endchildpoverty.org.uk** for more information.

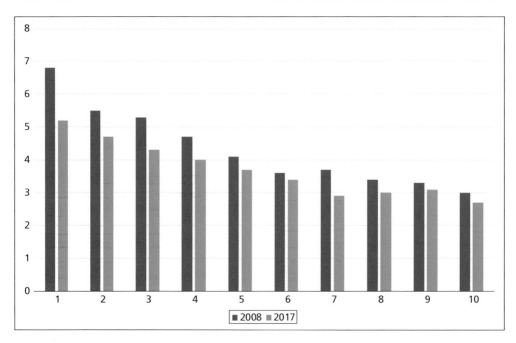

Figure 1.7 Infant mortality rates for most and least deprived areas in England, 2008 and 2017. Infant mortality rates are shown for the 10 deciles of the Index of Multiple Deprivation (1 is the most deprived, 10 is the least). *Source:* "Child and infant mortality in England and Wales: 2017", www.ons.gov.uk. Licensed under Open Government License v3.0.

children living in poverty has increased substantially over the last few decades to 30% (over four million children).

1.4.2 Changes in family structure

Family structure has become more fluid in the UK, reflecting changing societal attitudes to marriage, divorce and cohabitation. Children more often have to make transitions to new family structures. They are helped by: family stability; good relationships between partners; avoiding sustained exposure to conflict; and keeping children's needs paramount. Although marriage has declined and nearly 50% of births are now outside marriage, 7 out of 10 families are headed by a married or civil partner couple. Cohabiting couple families are increasing, along with step-family combinations. With more lone-parent families and families where both parents work, grandparents play a significant role in childcare (at least weekly for 25% of families); 22% of dependent children live in lone-parent families. Although UK teenage pregnancy rates have fallen recently, they are still among the highest across developed countries. Half of all teenage mothers live in the 20% most deprived areas.

Home factors that can adversely affect children's health and development include:

- Parental discord
  - Quarrelling
  - Separation and divorce
  - Domestic violence
- Parental illness
  - Death of a parent
  - Chronic disability
  - Physical illness
  - Mental illness
- Inability to cope with demands of parenting
- Abuse
- Financial hardship.

The complexity and multiplicity of the factors that cause a child to be disadvantaged sometimes make us feel helpless. However, since adversities compound one another, much may be achieved by modifying even one adverse factor.

Extensive medical and social services exist, particularly for handicapped children, but all too often they are best used by well-informed, middle-class parents, while the parents of the disadvantaged child do not use them sometimes because they do not know about them. All medical and paramedical staff have a duty to recognize children in need or in distress and to see that they benefit from the help that is available.

 KEY POINTS

All children need:
- Self-esteem (we need to feel wanted)
- At least one good human relationship (we need to trust and feel trusted)
- Firm supervision and clear boundaries (we need rules).

A small change that helps to achieve one of these for a child may make a big difference.

Twenty percent of the world's population live in absolute poverty. Nearly half of them are children.

1.4.3 Ethnicity

Most countries have ethnic minority communities with particular needs. The UK continues to become more ethnically diverse. In the UK, 15% of the population (and one-third of newborns) are from ethnic minority groups. There is great regional variation. Consanguinity (marrying a blood relative) is more common in some cultures (e.g. some Muslim communities), increasing the risk of recessively inherited disease. Rickets is more common in some ethnic groups due to diet, pigmented skin and lack of exposure to sunlight. There remain significant health inequalities for many minority groups in Europe.

Find out about your own local situation and be aware of cultural and health differences. These range from what names to use, through to differences in patterns of disease, through travel (e.g. malaria), contact (e.g. tuberculosis) or racial susceptibility (e.g. sickle cell disease). Understanding the importance of racial background, family, cultural and religious beliefs improves paediatric care.

Ethnic composition (2011) – England and Wales

White	86%
Asian/Asian British	7.5%
Black/Black British	3.3%
Mixed	2.2%
Other	1%

1.4.4   Laws relating to the young

For legal and safeguarding purposes, a child remains a 'child' up to the age of 18. However, many laws become operative at other ages. School education is compulsory for children aged 5 and over.

Children under 10 (under 8 in Scotland) are not considered 'criminally responsible' for their misdeeds and may be dealt with by youth courts. The court can make (1) a care order giving parental rights to the local authority; or (2) a supervision order which may be administered by the social services department or, if the child is over 14, by the probation department. At the age of 15, children can be sent to youth custody.

Adult courts deal with those over the age of 17. Although it is legally possible to be sent to prison for a first offence at the age of 17, in practice it is rare before the age of 20.

1.4.5   Ethics and children's rights

In 1989, the United Nations declared that children worldwide should have special rights due to their immaturity and vulnerability. This Convention on the Rights of the Child sets out what every child needs for 'a safe, happy and fulfilled childhood'. These include the right to health, family life and to have his views taken seriously in matters affecting him. Consent and competence are covered later (Section 17.2). Once a child is deemed to be competent, then the doctor has the normal duty of confidentiality, including not disclosing information to a third party (including a parent). Sometimes, this has to be overridden because of safeguarding concerns, but this should be explained to the child.

Decisions about when to limit treatment

Situations where the withholding or withdrawal of life-prolonging treatment **might** be considered:
- Life limited in quantity – treatment unable or unlikely to prolong life significantly (including when death is imminent or inevitable, or in brain stem death);
- Life limited in quality – although treatment may prolong life, the burden of the underlying condition, or of the treatment, may be too great;
- Informed competent refusal of treatment – particularly where young people have capacity and parents and clinical team support the decision.
  See the RCPCH Framework for Practice for more detailed discussion: https://bit.ly/2vJ5clH or via the RCPCH website www.rcpch.ac.uk.

A challenging part of intensive care (whether paediatric or neonatal) – and which sometimes makes headlines in the media – is the decision to withdraw life-prolonging treatment. Decisions should be made by the treating team in partnership with the parents, taking time to ensure all relevant information is considered, and what is in the best interests of the child.

1.5   Child health in the community

1.5.1   Health personnel

1.5.1.1   Community paediatricians

Most paediatricians have a commitment to some services outside of the hospital. Community paediatricians specialize in working outside of the hospital. They work closely with health visitors and the staff of child health clinics, and also with GPs, social and educational services. The boundary between hospital general paediatrics and community paediatrics is increasingly blurred. Community paediatricians often specialize in one or more of the following:

- Child health surveillance
- Provision of children's services to a specific geographical sector
- Learning problems and disability
- Child protection (child abuse)
- Audiology
- Adoption and fostering
- School health.

1.5.1.2   Health visitors (0–5 years)

These are registered nurses with additional training in health promotion and prevention of illness in all age groups. Many are attached to general practices and a few specialize (e.g. in diabetes) and have hospital attachments. They are responsible for family health and particularly for mothers and preschool children. Their job is to prevent illness and handicap by giving appropriate advice, by detecting problems early and by mobilizing services to deal with those problems. They have a key role in child health promotion.

1.5.1.3   School nurses (5–19 years)

School nurses provide a variety of school-based services:

- Confidential health advice for children and young people

> **Children Acts 1989 and 2004**
>
> The 1989 Act covered all aspects of the welfare and protection of children including day-care, fostering and adoption, child abuse and the consequences for children of marital breakdown. The spirit of the Act is reflected in the opening paragraphs:
>   'the child's welfare shall be the court's paramount consideration'
>   'any delay in determining the question (of the child's upbringing) is likely to prejudice the welfare of the child'
>   'a court shall have regard to … the ascertainable wishes and feelings of the child concerned'.
> The 2004 Act further developed the 1989 Act to improve child well-being and safety, including creation of a Children's Commissioner.
>   Both emphasize that all people and organizations who work with children have a responsibility for their safeguarding and well-being.

1.6.3   Voluntary services

The statutory services are supplemented by a large number of voluntary and charitable organizations, many of which were in existence before, and paved the way for, statutory provisions. Many of those offering services to children have a high level of professional expertise. The NSPCC (National Society for the Prevention of Cruelty to Children) and its Scottish counterpart continue their historic role of protecting children, and giving advice and support to families under stress. Barnardo's, the Children's Society and the National Children's Homes have adapted their activities to the changing pattern of child needs. The Save the Children Fund gives support to deprived inner cities in the UK as well as relief in developing countries. Many voluntary bodies receive some funding from central and/or local government.

1.6.3.1   Parent support groups

These exist for almost every chronic disorder of childhood (e.g. Cystic Fibrosis Trust). Their membership consists largely of parents of affected children who can offer advice to others from first-hand experience. They also raise money to support research, thereby augmenting the work of the major medical research charities.

1.6.3.2   The family fund

This gives financial help to less well-off families with very severely handicapped children. It is financed by the Department of Health, but administered by the Rowntree Trust in York. Charitable organizations can often minimize bureaucracy and cut administrative costs and delays.

1.6.4   Adoption

Couples wishing to adopt a child approach their local authority who will assess suitability. The process includes medical assessment of the child and parents. Once adopted, the child is a full member of the family; he or she takes their name and has all the rights of a natural child. It is best for parents to inform their child from the beginning that they are adopted.

1.7   Children in hospital

Health care for children has changed dramatically in the last 70 years. Children were separated from their parents for long periods with little appreciation of their particular needs. The birth and development of paediatrics as a medical specialty were largely attributable to the first children's hospitals. Now, the special needs of children are recognized in the design and provision of services, e.g. unrestricted visiting, facilities for resident parents, play activities for younger children (Figure 1.9) and education for older children. Every effort is made to minimize a child's need to stay in hospital, including ambulatory care (where care traditionally provided in hospital is moved to a home-based model). This may include short-stay assessment units and outreach nursing. Infants account for nearly half of all paediatric admissions (Figure 1.10). The majority of admissions

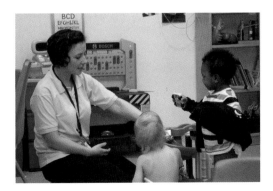

Figure 1.9 Children in hospital. The play specialist plays a vital role.

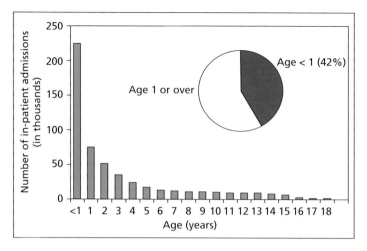

Figure 1.10 Number of paediatric in-patient admissions by age. Number of admissions per year in 1000s in the UK of children 0–18 years old. *Source:* Audit Commission 1993. Public Domain.

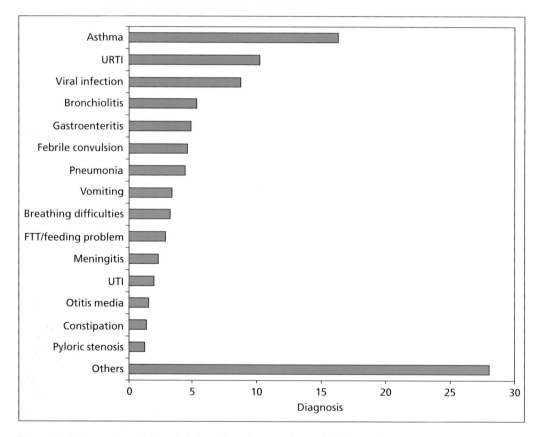

Figure 1.11 Causes of paediatric admissions. Based on a study of admissions to a District General Hospital. Respiratory problems (asthma, URTI, bronchiolitis, pneumonia and breathing difficulties) caused 57% of admissions, and infective illness 44%. FTT, failure to thrive; URTI, upper respiratory tract infection; UTI, urinary tract infection. *Source:* Based on Thakker, Y., Sheldon, T. A., Long, R., and MacFaul, R. (1994). Paediatric inpatient utilisation in a district general hospital. *Archives of Disease in Childhood* 70(6): 488–492. doi:10.1136/adc.70.6.488.

are due to respiratory conditions and infections (Figure 1.11).

PRACTICE POINT   Infection control

Make sure you know and adhere to hand hygiene and other infection control guidance during your paediatric placement. This will not only protect children on the wards from cross-infection, but protect you too!

Hospitals are not without risk to patients, especially child patients. The hazard of cross-infection is obvious: the hazard of mother–child separation is less obvious but can be more serious, especially among the 1- to 4-year-olds. At this age, children are old enough to grieve for a lost mother, but not old enough to understand the reason, or that the separation is temporary. 'Tomorrow' has no meaning for a toddler.

PRACTICE POINT   Patient safety

As in the rest of medicine, recognition of the potential for the process of care to cause harm has led to initiatives to make care safer. Some issues are the same as in adult care (for instance miscommunication, surgical process), while others are peculiar to paediatrics, such as certain prescribing challenges (Chapter 30), non-specific symptomatology in young children, who may suddenly 'crash'. Paediatric patient safety initiatives include:
- Paediatric early warning score charts – these empower all involved to seek early review for patients who are deteriorating
- Safety 'huddles' to highlight particular ward issues
- Handover protocols to clearly identify ill patients, those with similar names, and those with safeguarding issues
- Drug prescribing – checks by pharmacists, alerts built into electronic systems
- Drug administration – e.g. nurses wearing red apron during this task are not disturbed
- Safety netting advice to parents on discharge
- Procedure checklists
- Quality improvement and learning culture; learning from adverse events and 'near – misses'.

Changes in hospital care
- The average stay in hospital is much shorter.
- There are similar numbers of medical and surgical admissions.
- More children are admitted – 1 in 4 by age 2 years, 1 in 3 by 4.5 years.
- Many medical and surgical procedures are done as day cases.
- Parents are actively involved in care.
- Outreach nursing teams and day assessment units reduce the need for admission.
- Neonatal care makes increasingly heavy demands on resources.

A young child separated from his mother may go through three stages:

Protest: he cries for her return.

Withdrawal: he curls up with a comfort blanket or toy and loses interest in food and play.

Denial: he appears happy, making indiscriminate friendships with everybody. This can be mistakenly interpreted as the child having 'settled', but the mother–child bond has been damaged and will have to be rebuilt. On returning home, he may exhibit tantrums, refuse food or wet his bed.

These problems can be avoided or minimized by:

- Avoiding hospital admission if possible
- Reducing the length of any admission to the minimum
- Performing operations (e.g. herniotomy, orchidopexy) and investigations (e.g. jejunal biopsy, colonoscopy) as day cases
- Encouraging parents to visit often and arranging for one to sleep alongside a young child.

Hospital organization can also help to reduce stress. Paediatric wards mean that children are looked after by staff specially trained and experienced in the care of children in a child-friendly environment. Teachers, nursery nurses and play leaders organize education and play. The first impression of a children's ward should be of happy chaos, rather than of the highly technical medicine, which is in fact going on.

1.8 Research and evidence-based medicine

Many of the remarkable improvements in health outcomes for children that you will read about in this book are due to research discoveries which have been implemented through an evidence-based medicine approach. No longer is it sufficient to adapt research in adult patients and treatments to children, whose conditions may have quite different underlying pathophysiology. Research networks, international collaborations and multicenter trials enable advances in care even in rare conditions. Follow the 'Research Trail' boxes in this book for a tour of some of the key research that has improved child health, primarily over the last 50 years. Perhaps you will make a contribution in the next 50...?

 Research Trail:
Examples of research that have transformed child health

- The extended immunization programme has contributed to the global improvement in child mortality
- Infants put to sleep on their backs has hugely reduced SIDS
- Improvement in childhood cancer outcomes through multicenter trials, e.g. survival rates for acute lymphoblastic leukaemia have risen from around 20% to over 90%
- Cystic fibrosis care is on the verge of a new era due to new drugs that work on the membrane transporter protein
- Spina bifida is rare due to the discovery that folic acid supplementation in pregnancy prevents it
- Surfactant has transformed outcomes for preterm babies
- Prevention of HIV transmission from mother to baby has greatly improved outcomes
- Insulin therapy has revolutionized management of diabetes, and closed loop pumps are now in clinical use

Next Research Trail on page 70

 # Summary

Although most of this book will focus on illness and disease in children, the issues we have covered in this chapter are vital to understanding child health and need to underpin all your work with children and families. Most of the global burden of childhood disease is in developing countries, and the good news is that progress is being made to reduce this. Health inequalities are important to UK child health – if poverty could be eradicated, more than 1000 child deaths each year would be prevented. Health promotion is of great importance, as are the social aspects of child health. When you meet children and their families in hospital, a thoughtful, sensitive and child-friendly approach can transform a 'job to be done' into a positive and even therapeutic encounter.

 FOR YOUR LOG

- Find out about child health statistics for your local area – in the UK go to https://fingertips.phe.org.uk and explore the child health profiles and data atlas.
- Discuss local child health issues with paediatric (and if accessible) public health staff.
- Look up parent support group websites for some of the conditions you come across – *Contact a family* is a good place to start (www.contact.org.uk).
- Visit a preschool or school catering for children with special health or learning needs if this can be organized within your course.
- Visit community health facilities and primary care – focusing on provision for children.
- Follow the 'Research Trail' in this book, and find out about local paediatric research.

2

Parents and children: listening and talking

Chapter map

You will have already learnt the importance of good communication skills in adult medicine. In paediatrics, you need to extend and develop these skills, not only so that you can take an effective history, but so that you can conduct a whole consultation with children and parents together, reassure appropriately and break difficult news. This chapter will focus on history taking, but will also cover some wider aspects of communication.

2.1   History taking and diagnosis

 Paediatric history taking is vital because it usually holds the key to the diagnosis.

Diagnosis involves a recurring cycle where you formulate and test hypotheses. As you collect more information about the patient, you will reject some diagnoses and come up with alternatives that were not on your original list (Figure 2.1). When you first begin paediatrics, it is useful to work through a list of standard questions. Once you are familiar with these, aim to move towards problem-orientated histories: generate mental lists of differentials for common presenting symptoms and then focus your history around these. This thoughtful, logical approach is much better than blindly asking a series of questions that you have learned by rote.

 Your goal is to be able to come up with appropriate differential diagnoses for common and important paediatric presentations. This underpins good history taking. Use the symptom sorter (p. 370) and text of this book to help you.

Paediatrics Lecture Notes, Tenth Edition. Jonathan C. Darling and James Yong.
© 2022 John Wiley & Sons Ltd. Published 2022 by John Wiley & Sons Ltd.
Companion website: www.wiley.com/go/lecturenotes/paediatrics10e

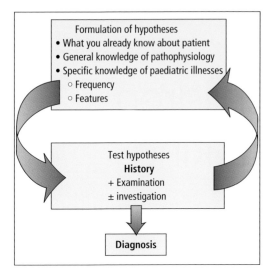

Figure 2.1 Reaching a diagnosis. It is important to start with a reasonable differential diagnosis (your hypotheses). The 'Symptom sorter' in this book can help. The history contributes much more than examination or investigations.

Differences from an adult history

Triadic consultation: the child, their family and the doctor

Indirect information from parents

Child's contribution important but variable and unpredictable

Different elements of history
- perinatal and birth
- development
- immunization
- family and social history emphasis

Different illnesses and time courses

Need to adapt to child's age and development

Possibility of child abuse

Adolescents need a different approach (see Chapter 17).

2.1.1 Parents

Throughout most of childhood, parents act as the child's advocate and interpreter. Parents tell us about the child's symptoms – although the children contribute more and more as they grow older.

Parents put into effect any treatments needed outside hospital.

Small children only survive because their parents are concerned about them. A few are less concerned than they should be, and their children suffer from neglect. Others are more than usually concerned. Do not regard overanxious parents as a nuisance. Instead, view their genuine concern for their child positively and help them cope with their anxieties through patient reassurance.

> 🔑 Beware of accepting parents' **interpretations** of their child's behaviour at face value. Ask 'What exactly did you see that made you think that?' (Table 2.1).

Table 2.1 Fact and interpretation in history and examination

Fact	Interpretation
She cries and draws her legs up to her tummy	Our baby has colic
He has watery stools six times a day, whereas his normal stool is formed and once daily	He has bad diarrhoea
She gets wheezy when she runs	She has asthma
He falls asleep at school	He is lazy at school

2.1.2 Involving the child

Children from about 2 years can hear, understand and say a lot. By 7 or 8 years, they are wise. Do not talk about them as if they had no understanding – and you may have to discourage parents from doing the same. Sometimes, if both are agreeable, it is useful to talk to the parent(s) and the child privately to allow them to express concerns or to give particular advice. Older teenagers may prefer to be seen on their own first. Whatever the medical problem, the child is first a child. Not 'he is a diabetic' or 'she is an epileptic': he has diabetes, she has epilepsy.

2.1.3 History taking

The child's history covers the same ground as that of an adult patient, with some important additions.

Standard paediatric history

(additions to adult history in italics – can be summarized under acronym BINDS)
Name/Age/Sex/Consultant/*Historian*
Presenting complaint
History of presenting complaint
Past medical history
- **B***irth and neonatal history*
  - *Where*
  - *Delivery*
  - *Gestation*
  - *Weight*
  - *Ante/postnatal problems*
  - *Neonatal problems (jaundice, SCBU, ventilation, antibiotics)*
  - *Maternal health*
- **I***mmunizations*
- **N***utrition and Feeding – neonatal, weaning, concerns about growth*
- **D***evelopment*

Illnesses, operations and accidents
Drugs
Allergies
Family and **S***ocial history*
- *Mother – name/age/occupation/health*
- *Father – name/age/occupation/health*
- *Siblings – name/age/health*
- *Inherited or genetic conditions*
- *Contact with common infections*
- *Nursery/school*
- *Pets*
- *Housing.*

2.1.3.1 Approach

- Address the parents by name, not as 'mum' or 'dad'
- Find out what the child is called at home and use that name
- Begin your notes with the name, sex and the age in years and months – accurate age is essential and often defines the differential diagnosis
- Note the name of the school, nursery, clinic or health centre she attends
- Consider the child during the history
  - a young child may be happiest on a parent's knee
  - a more independent one may prefer playing with toys, which should be available
  - an older child must be fully included in the discussion
- Arrange the furniture to encourage a sense of partnership between parents and doctor and avoid confrontation over the top of a desk.

 PRACTICE POINT

If the parents do not speak English, insist on an interpreter. Do not try to use the child as an interpreter, except in emergencies.

2.1.3.2 History of the presenting condition

Begin with this, because it is what they have come to tell you about. Let them tell it their own way first; then ask specific questions to fill in necessary details (Figure 2.2). Frequent interruptions or insistence on ordered chronology inhibit free speech.

 PRACTICE POINT

- Start with OPEN questions: How is she? Why are you worried?
- Add CLOSED questions: How often does he wheeze? Which inhaler do you use most?

Ask about patterns of eating, sleeping and activity. If these have not changed, serious illness is unlikely. A reduction in appetite or activity, or an increased need for sleep, is likely to be significant. Recorded weight loss is always important.

 PRACTICE POINT

- Always find out how the illness affects the child's life
- Normal activity, e.g. does acute asthma stop the child from running, walking and talking?
- School – for non-acute problems, how much school has been missed through illness?
- Social – is the child opting out of games or of leisure activities at home?

What are the parents' own ideas about what is the matter with the child? Sometimes this will alert you to an unnecessary anxiety; at other times, it may lead to a correct diagnosis you had not considered. Mothers are more likely than anyone else to understand their babies' cries, and research shows that babies can 'talk'. They have different cries for

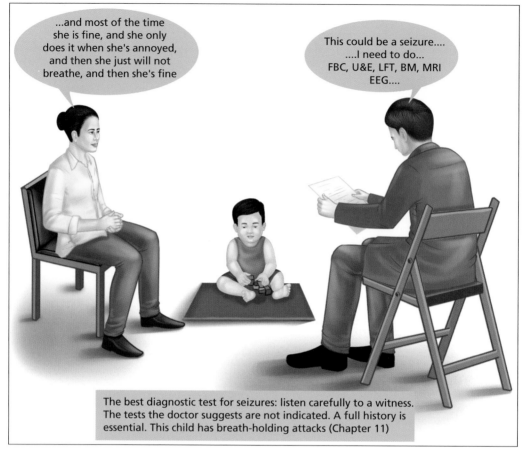

Figure 2.2 The best diagnostic test for seizures is a good history.

hunger, pain, etc. The mother will usually know when the cry is abnormal and sometimes will be able to suggest a reason.

It is often helpful, especially if psychological problems are suspected, to ask 'What kind of boy is he?' The answer may be 'a worrier', 'placid', 'never still', 'obsessional'. If you then ask 'Who does he take after?', it often provides useful insight for the parent. It is also helpful to know what the child does in his spare time and whether he is by nature gregarious or solitary.

PRACTICE POINT

Make a note of who gave you the history, who referred and location.

> **? OSCE Pointer**
>
> Students often move on from the presenting complaint too quickly. Make sure you have understood precisely what is happening, impact on child and family, and details of any previous treatment (including name, dose, when given and by whom and effect).

2.1.3.3 Previous medical history – pointers

- Immunization history: it may help to exclude a suspected condition, and it identifies those families in need of advice about further immunization.
- Ask the parents for the personal child health record (and thank them for having brought it) (Figure 1.8).

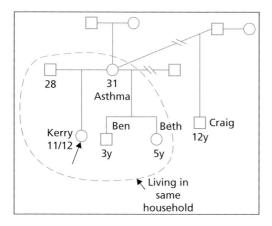

Figure 2.3 Family tree. The broken lines between parents indicate a separation. Ben and Beth live in the same household as Kerry (who is the presenting child, indicated with an arrow), but are her half-siblings, to mother's previous partner.

This includes details of previous weights, immunizations and other health events.

2.1.3.4 Family history – pointers

- The ages of the siblings and parents (usefully noted on a family tree, Figure 2.3).
- Whether any other member of the family has had the same condition as the child
  - e.g. a rash and fever (has the child caught the same infection?)
  - e.g. six digits on each hand (an inherited condition).
- What illnesses the parents and close relatives have had, in order to identify familial and infective problems and allay needless worries. The parents may worry that their child's stomach ache is caused by stomach cancer, because a relative recently died with it.
- An enquiry regarding consanguinity, especially in suspected metabolic or inherited conditions, because these are more likely if the parents are related.

 PRACTICE POINT

Diagnostic signs on examination are rare; the child's diagnosis lies in the history.

2.1.3.5 Perinatal history

- Pregnancy
  - gestation (normal is 40 weeks)
- illnesses

- medications
- smoking and alcohol
- Delivery
  - place (hospital/home)
  - presentation (head/breech)
  - type (spontaneous, forceps, caesarean section)
- Birthweight
- Neonatal period
  - risk factors for neonatal sepsis (maternal Group B strep, premature rupture of membranes)
  - abnormalities
  - illnesses
  - need for special/intensive care
  - day of discharge home.

2.1.3.6 Developmental history

This is almost unique to paediatrics. It is important, particularly for young children, or where there is concern about disability or developmental delay. It includes details of the times at which skills such as walking and talking were acquired (Chapter 10).

2.1.3.7 Social history

After establishing rapport with the parents, talk with them about their life, their home, their work and their problems. Parental employment may give insight into particular pressures for the family and level of understanding of health issues. Who looks after the child if both parents work? If one parent is full time at home, what was their job before?

 PRACTICE POINT

Preface these questions with an explanation that an understanding of the child's home and family can often help with diagnosis and management. Ask sensitively. Otherwise, they can seem irrelevant or intrusive.

Explore the following areas, since they have a direct influence on the child:

- Family composition
  - other children in the home?
  - who are the main carers?
  - do parents live together?
  - other significant adults in the home or close to child (e.g. grandparents)
- Family pressures
  - what do parents see as stressful for themselves or their children?

- may include busy jobs, financial hardship, parental discord, neighbourhood harassment
- Housing
  - stability – frequent moves can be unsettling and affect the continuity of health care
  - space – cramped or overcrowded accommodation is stressful for all and increases infection transmission
  - specific needs – children with disability may need modifications to their home
  - difficulties – some families struggle with housing problems which dominate family life.

 PRACTICE POINT

Drawing out a family tree with the parents' help is a good way to understand family arrangements (Figure 2.3). This can be annotated with details of illnesses, names and dates (e.g. of bereavement/ separation/divorce).

2.2   The consultation

Families are often anxious on arrival, waiting for the doctor's 'verdict'. Their fears are often worse than the reality.

 PRACTICE POINT

Each person who sees the family should introduce themselves, explain their role and what they are going to do. This is essential to good care, but still omitted by many – see www.hellomynameis.org.uk.

As a student, you should check the parents are happy to speak to you, and clarify your task and the time available with the doctor supervising you. Once the history and examination have been completed, the remainder of the consultation often takes one of three directions:

- Explanation and reassurance
- Investigation and/or treatment but with a favourable outcome probable
- Bad news.

Students may be involved in discussing aspects of the first two under supervision, but should not attempt to break bad news. If a child or parent asks you questions, when you do not know the answer, admit it. Offer to find someone who can help.

2.2.1   Reassurance

- Readily accepted by some parents who 'just wanted to make sure everything was all right'.
- Remember that the presenting condition may only be a pretext to visit and that more serious concerns lie elsewhere.
- Some parents are very difficult to reassure
  - careful explanation is usually helpful – parents may stop worrying if they understand why the doctor is not worried.
  - a specific anxiety needs an equally specific reassurance, e.g. parents who fear their child's pallor is due to leukaemia may need to be told 'She has not got leukaemia', rather than just that the blood count is normal.

2.2.2   Investigations and treatments

- Explain honestly and in advance
  - don't say it won't hurt if it will – but you can emphasize the things that will minimize anything unpleasant.
  - an MRI scan is noisy (play specialists can help, but very young children, may require a general anaesthetic).
- Give results promptly with clear explanation and interpretation
  - parents appreciate being told the results of tests, and their implications, promptly – a phone call often helps.
- Explain and give reasons for treatments
  - some treatments are flexible and others not, and it helps if parents understand the rationale, e.g. why four times a day?
  - demonstrate techniques for the use of inhalers for asthma, injections for diabetes or rectally administered anticonvulsants.

Parents are increasingly informed about health issues, through the internet, media and social media. Unfortunately, these tend to exaggerate or sensationalize, presenting an experimental new treatment as a 'breakthrough', or a particular clinic or hospital (often in another country) as 'the only one of its kind' and hence, by implication, the best. It may be an uphill task to put things in perspective. We need special understanding for parents who have been offered hope when they had none before.

2.2.3   Bad news

This usually concerns:

- a birth defect in a newborn baby
- a serious handicap in a young child

- a serious, progressive or incurable disease
- safeguarding concerns (see Chapter 16).

The news that a baby is abnormal is a great shock to the parents. Even minor anomalies are seen as major tragedies. At the first interview, detailed explanations will not be grasped. Later, parents will need detailed explanation of the care needed and how to recognize any problems that are likely to arise.

PRACTICE POINT

Parents want to know:
- Exactly what is the matter, in terms they can grasp
- What the doctors can do about it
- What the parents can do about it
- The outlook for this child
- The outlook for any other children that may follow
- Why it happened (did they cause it?).

2.2.3.1 Breaking bad news

- Both parents present if possible
- Unhurried (no bleeps)
- Consider whether child or young person should be present
- Ask what the parents understand
- Clear information
- Diagrams and/or printed materials for reference
- Regularly summarize and invite questions
- Make a clear plan.

Parents' self-help groups can provide information, leaflets and mutual support. Parents should be told about them.

PRACTICE POINT

When transferring a baby to another hospital (e.g. for surgery, neonatal intensive care)
- Ensure the parents see their infant before transfer
- Arrange frequent progress reports until mother is able to visit.

2.2.3.2 Genetic counselling

Parents of children with serious defects or handicaps need advice about the recurrence risks if they plan another child later on. For easily recognisable conditions in which a genetic (or non-genetic) basis is clearly established, the family doctor or paediatrician can provide this information. For more complex problems, refer to a *genetic counselling* clinic.

Essentials of genetic counselling
- A firmly established diagnosis (often more difficult than it sounds)
- Knowledge of inheritance
- A full family history
- Ample time to elicit facts and anxieties, and to explain recurrence risks, prenatal tests and other relevant issues.

2.2.3.3 Parents' reactions to bad news (Figure 2.4)

- Recognizable pattern
- Time scale varies widely from one family to another
- Important for doctors to recognize this pattern
  - to help the family
  - to understand parents' negative reactions (e.g. anger towards the doctor).
- The stages of adaptation to personal tragedy, which often overlap, are as follows:
1 Intellectual and emotional numbness
  - Information does not get in, emotions do not get out.
    - health staff may be relieved that the parents have 'taken it so well'
    - don't be annoyed if parents later say 'nobody told us anything' when you spent hours telling them everything.
2 Denial
  - The message has got through but cannot yet be believed.
    - e.g. 'There must be some mistake' or 'But he will catch up, won't he?'
  - Resist the temptation to hedge or use woolly phrases (e.g. 'slow developer') – they may falsely encourage parents to believe that the problem is curable.
3 Guilt and anger
  - The truth has registered and blame must be apportioned.
    - parents often blame themselves – for some act of commission or omission, real or imaginary

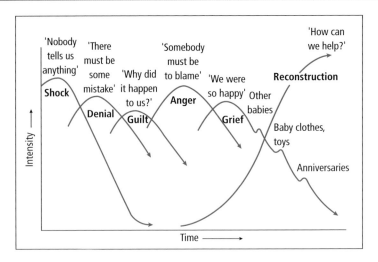

Figure 2.4 Emotional response to bad news.

○ blame others – the feeling of guilt may be so intolerable that the parents blame someone else (the doctor) or something else (the treatment).

4 Grief
- A natural and healing process.
- Tears are healthy – the health professional who shares these moments should feel privileged, not embarrassed.

5 Reconstruction
- The former pattern of family life has been demolished; the new must now be built.
- Give parents a key, active role in any therapeutic programme.
- Never say 'Nothing can be done' – it is not true.

aware of the possibility of child abuse. There is no substitute for practice, and we hope you will enjoy taking and presenting many paediatric histories and reviewing them with your teachers.

 FOR YOUR LOG

Summarizing a history is key clinical skill. Write a brief (2–3 sentence) summary for every history you take. The process clarifies what is important in your mind, makes your verbal presentation clearer and means you finish neatly. OSCE stations involving history taking or presentation will often ask for a summary.

 Summary

We have described how the paediatric history and consultation differs from adult medicine. There are different elements (such as birth, immunizations, development), but more importantly there is a different approach. This includes involving the child according to age, understanding the constraints of working through a third party (the parent) and being

 OSCE pointers

- History of any common presenting symptom or problem.
- Counselling and explaining common and important paediatric problems, e.g. constipation, weaning, immunization, gastro-oesophageal reflux, asthma, febrile convulsions, epilepsy, enuresis. Avoid jargon!

OSCE station 2.1: Counselling

Clinical approach:
- Read any facts given to you
- Have mental/written list of main points
- Ask open questions at beginning and end (e.g. is there anything else you would like me to talk about?)
- Note reasons for special concern (e.g. other member of family with same problem)
- Deal with common concerns
- Remember body language – yours and the mother's
- Listen
- It may help to write down the diagnosis or draw a diagram.

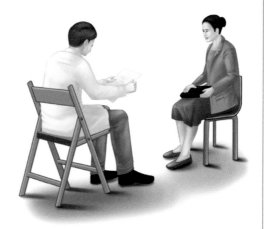

Information to give
- Diagnosis, description of problem
- What do we know?
- The cause
- Explain the child's symptoms
- What can be done?
- How will it affect the child?
- What treatment?
- What investigations?
- Follow-up

Never forget:
- Say hello and introduce yourself
- General health – is the child ill?
- Empathic enquiry: how is Sally today?
- Are you and the child's parent comfortable?

Look around for:
- Hospital records
- Information leaflets

Special points
- In some examinations, you will be given a history first
- Listen for hints to unexpressed worries

Please talk to this mother. Her 3-year-old son had a febrile convulsion 2 days ago and is now well. She would like to discuss this with you before going home
- Listen to what she knows
- Explain diagnosis
  - ◇ Fit caused by fever in healthy child
  - ◇ 6 months – 5 years of age
- Common (3% of all children)
- Fits are frightening but seldom dangerous
  - ◇ How did parents feel during child's fit?
  - ◇ Many parents think that their child is dying
- Prognosis good
  - ◇ Most have no more febrile fits
  - ◇ One-third will have a second episode
  - ◇ Epilepsy rare
- Prevention
  - ◇ Recognition of fever
  - ◇ Light clothing
  - ◇ Antipyretics do not prevent further convulsions and should only be used for distress
- Further fits
  - ◇ First aid
  - ◇ When to seek help

*'Parent' may be a trained actor or a member of staff
The child is not present*

3

Examination of children

Chapter map

Examining children, especially the very young, seems daunting at first, but most children are cooperative, and clinical examination should be a happy experience for them. Children are usually accompanied by a parent, who will help you, and appreciate being involved. This chapter assumes you are already competent to do systems examinations in adult patients. We will show you how to adjust your examination according to the child's age, show you how to approach any clinical examination of a child and emphasize key differences in paediatric examination, including attention to growth, nutrition and pubertal status.

The obvious reason for examination is to find abnormal signs that help make the diagnosis. In acute illness, symptoms are often non-specific. The general impression of a child's health is all important. You will miss essential signs (e.g. infected throat, stiff neck or infected urine) if you do not look for them systematically. In chronic illness, subtle signs can be clues to the diagnosis. For example, minor congenital abnormalities or dysmorphic features can point to a syndrome, or chronic chest deformity or clubbing may indicate chronic respiratory disease. Assessment of growth is always helpful. Parents and children often come to the paediatrician concerned about severe disease. A 'thorough examination' is a powerful therapeutic weapon in the face of parental anxiety. Parents do not readily accept reassurance from the doctor who has not examined the child – and quite right too!

Paediatrics Lecture Notes, Tenth Edition. Jonathan C. Darling and James Yong.
© 2022 John Wiley & Sons Ltd. Published 2022 by John Wiley & Sons Ltd.
Companion website: www.wiley.com/go/lecturenotes/paediatrics10e

PRACTICE POINT **Chaperones**

As a student, you should not perform sensitive or intimate examinations that might cause a child or adolescent embarrassment. As a doctor, request a chaperone at these times.

 PRACTICE POINT **Age-specific approach to examining children**

- *Newborn infants*: in the early weeks of life, patience, warm hands and a quiet voice are needed. Bedside manner contributes little (but is important to parents).
- *2–10 months*: infants respond to the friendly doctor, and examination is often easy if the child is generally comfortable. A smiling face can evoke rapport and even cooperation.
- *10 months–5 years*: toddlers present the biggest challenge. The toddler is generally suspicious of strangers. Their confidence must be won, perhaps by giving them something to hold, or taking interest in their toy. An unhurried, confident approach is most likely to lead to success. Young children do not like to be separated from their parents, rapidly undressed or made to lie flat. Examine the child on their parent's knee rather than an examination couch. Be patient and adapt the pace and the order of the examination to the child's level of comfort and confidence.
- *5–10 years*: school-age children are used to being without their parents, but still want them close by in unfamiliar surroundings. They are generally cooperative. They enjoy neurological examination and like to listen to their heart through a stethoscope. A worried child can be diverted by chatting to them.
- *10 years to teenage*: the process of examining the older child and teenager is usually straightforward. Cooperation is almost guaranteed if the doctor respects their independence, maturity and modesty. Ask them whether they would prefer their parents to be present and seek their permission to examine them. Often the history taking will be dominated by a parent, and most teenagers cannot tell you their birthweight! The time of the examination is an opportunity to talk to the older child about their perspective and concerns.

3.1 A system of examination

In acute paediatrics, outpatients and in undergraduate examinations, the clinical examination begins with general assessment and then moves on to look at specific systems. All who are new to paediatrics must begin by learning these skills.

 PRACTICE POINT

Watch paediatricians closely to pick up ideas to add to your own repertoire of ways to help children feel at ease.

A good history will raise specific questions, e.g. this history could be pneumonia. Is this child unwell? Is she tachypnoeic or febrile?

3.1.1 Initial assessment

Clinical examination has certain essential elements; these are made during the first approach to the child and should be carefully recorded. The most striking finding in a young child with pneumonia, for example, is that they appear ill. The positive clinical findings of lobar consolidation are difficult to elicit and may be absent.

3.1.2 HIGHCOST

This acronym emphasizes the importance of the first clinical impression and simple observation, which are central to good paediatric clinical assessment. It might also remind you that good clinical assessment is expensive of time, but highly cost-effective! It is a useful approach to systems examination in the Objective Structured Clinical Examination (OSCE) (Chapter 29).

Hello
Introduce yourself
General inspection
Health and hands
Centiles
Obvious
Systems examination
Thank you

3.1.3 Hello

Children are quick to assess adults and often very accurate. Approach the child with courtesy, a smile and a friendly greeting. There are two essential reasons that every undergraduate should remember this: it is an important clinical skill, and in almost every OSCE you will get marks for it!

3.1.4 Introduce yourself

Introduce yourself and find out to whom you are speaking. What does the child like to be called? Matt may only be called Matthew when his parents are annoyed with him.

RESOURCE

The importance of introducing yourself is well made by the 'Hello my name is. . .' campaign **www. hellomynameis.org.uk**

3.1.5 General inspection

During the general introduction, and often while taking the clinical history, you will learn a lot about the child, her parents and the relationships between them. You should also note if the child has an unusual appearance or abnormal features which fit into a recognized pattern (e.g. Down syndrome, achondroplasia).

PRACTICE POINT

Do not tower over the child, or lean over them during examination, but get down to their level.

Note the following:

- Does the child look well cared for? (Be careful – some clean, well-behaved children are unloved, while some caring parents may not see hygiene and clothing as a priority.)
- Is there a loving relationship between the child and the parents? Do the parents talk as if the child were not there, or as if she is an inanimate object? Are the parents showing an appropriate level of concern while sharing the problem with you?
- Is the child confident or clinging to the parent? Is he crying? When he seeks reassurance from his parent, does he get it? These are difficult assessments, particularly when a child is unwell.

- Does the child have any unusual features? Are the body proportions appropriate? Look at the child's face. Before you decide a child is dysmorphic, look at the parents' faces.

Dysmorphic features

These refer to variations in appearance or body structure that may be normal, but when several cluster together may indicate an underlying syndrome. Individuals with the same syndrome may share a similar appearance, rather like a family resemblance. Centile charts are available for most body measurements and variations in childhood. It is helpful to know some terms:

- Hypertelorism – widely spaced eyes (hypotelorism – eyes close together)
- Palpebral fissures the space between the eyelids, normally horizontal, may be slanted
- Epicanthic folds – fold of skin from upper lid covering inner canthus (corner) of the eye
- Philtrum – the vertical groove between the nose and upper lip (e.g. flattened or smooth in foetal alcohol syndrome)
- Brachycephaly – flattened occiput
- Clinodactyly – curved finger

3.1.6 Health and hands

- Is the child ill or well? Ask yourself this question every time you examine a child.
- In the young child, this is often the most important clinical sign. In the acutely unwell, 6-month-old infant, a pale, listless unresponsive appearance with glazed eyes has essential implications for diagnosis and immediate management. The experienced parent who simply reports that their child is ill should be listened to carefully.

 Children can change very quickly. A child who was satisfactory at triage may be moribund an hour later. If in doubt, don't press on with your assessment but call a member of staff.

Facial appearance may be helpful. Look for swelling, pallor, jaundice or cyanosis and assess hydration (see Table 22.2). Jaundice may be difficult to detect in artificial light. Examine the palpebral conjunctiva for signs of anaemia (evert the lower eyelid).

PRACTICE POINT

A hospital doctor who receives a phone call from a GP stating that the diagnosis is not clear, but that the child looks ill, should appreciate the urgency and importance of this statement.

Features that raise concern:

- a child who is inattentive, limp or intermittently distressed
- pallor, mottled skin or the infant who appears grey
- hypoxia may make a child sleepy or agitated
- cyanosis may be hard to see
- dehydration (Section 22.2.4.2)
- increased work of breathing (Section 3.5.3)
- fever, particularly if there is no clear cause.

It is often helpful to start the examination by holding the child's hand. It is not only a friendly gesture, but is often informative.

- Quickly assess the pulse. The radial pulse is commonly used, but in infants, the brachial may be easier to feel.
- Assess perfusion. Are the hands well-perfused or cold and clammy?
- Capillary refill is assessed by gently squeezing the nail so that the nail bed becomes pale. Upon release, the nail bed should again become pink within 2 s. Pale hands may indicate anaemia, which is better assessed from the conjunctiva.
- Look for clubbing. Although uncommon in children, when present it is an important physical sign.

3.1.7 Centiles

PRACTICE POINT

Assessment of growth is a fundamental part of paediatric examination (see below).

Although with experience you can make some assessment visually, you should always plot measurements on

OSCE TIP

In any paediatric OSCE station, consider including the following: *'I would like to assess growth by measuring height and weight, plotting on a centile chart, and comparing to previous measurements, if available'*. For an infant, include head circumference as well.

a centile chart. In an examination, saying that you would like to do this may be all that is necessary. If possible, compare with previous measurements in the parent-held record or the hospital notes. The trend of the plots is more important than their absolute positions.

3.1.8 Obvious

It is surprisingly easy to omit or even not notice the obvious, especially when you are focusing on a particular system, so include this as a deliberate step in your assessment. Often these observations give important clues to the diagnosis. Record or comment on the leg in plaster, the central venous line, the nasogastric tube, ankle/foot orthoses (splints) or a pile of inhalers. Record any injuries.

3.1.9 Systems examination

In paediatrics, each system does not need to be examined in a fixed order. Often examination of the body systems must be opportunistic. If the toddler is undressed and lying peacefully in his mother's arms, you might begin by listening to the heart. Leave potentially upsetting procedures (inspection of the throat) until last. Many children prefer not to be undressed completely, although by the end of examination all parts of the body should have been inspected. In undergraduate examination, genitalia should not be examined, except in young infants and rectal examination should never be performed. During systems examination, put the child at ease by asking about their family, friends, pets, hobbies or favourite TV programmes. Keep any instruments (tendon hammer, auroscope, etc.) out of sight until you need them, then show them to the child and explain how they work.

3.1.10 Thank you

Gratitude for the privilege of examining a child is never misplaced. The family will all appreciate praise for a child's good behaviour and cooperation.

OSCE TIP

In an examination, never do anything that is painful, likely to cause discomfort, or which is embarrassing. Some tasks are not practical or appropriate in the OSCE setting. If you are going to omit part of the examination for these reasons, explain this to the examiner (e.g. in the cardiac examination, say that you would want to: plot growth centiles, measure BP with correct cuff and examine femoral pulses).

3.2 Growth and nutrition

The characteristics of children which most clearly distinguish them from adults are growth (increase in size) and development (organ maturation, sexual development and the acquisition of new skills) (Figure 3.1).

 PRACTICE POINT

Plot with a single dot as accurately as you can – crosses and circles obscure subsequent plots. Use the chart already in the notes or in the parent held record (Figure 1.8). If you have to start a new one, label it.

3.2.1 Centile charts (Figure 3.2)

To assess growth, plot weight and height (and head circumference in infants, Figure 3.3) on centile charts. These are constructed from measurements of many children who are free from recognized problems which affect their growth. Children should be weighed either in underclothes (babies in nappies) or naked, but always the same way because changes in weight are more important than absolute values. Height is measured with a wall-mounted stadiometer, and you need tuition and practice to be able to do this accurately. For a child who is not yet walking, measure length supine on a horizontal stadiometer with a moveable foot board. Two people are needed to do this accurately. If children are upset at the prospect of being weighed and measured, postpone until the clinical examination is over: tears are more easily prevented than stopped.

 PRACTICE POINT

Remember to adjust plots for prematurity (i.e. less than 37 weeks of gestation) for the first year of life. A dotted horizontal arrow from the plot for the actual age to the one for the adjusted age makes the adjustment clear.

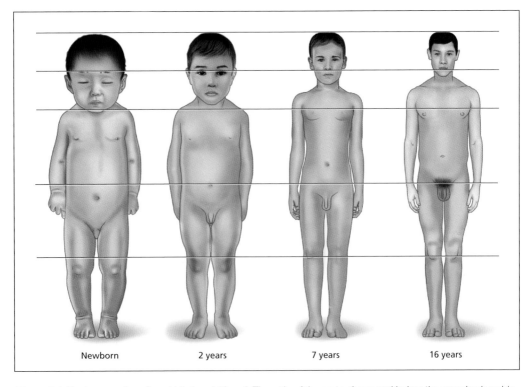

Newborn　　2 years　　7 years　　16 years

Figure 3.1 Body proportions from birth to adulthood. The ratio of the parts above and below the symphysis pubis falls from 1.7 : 1 in the newborn to 0.9 : 1 in the adult.

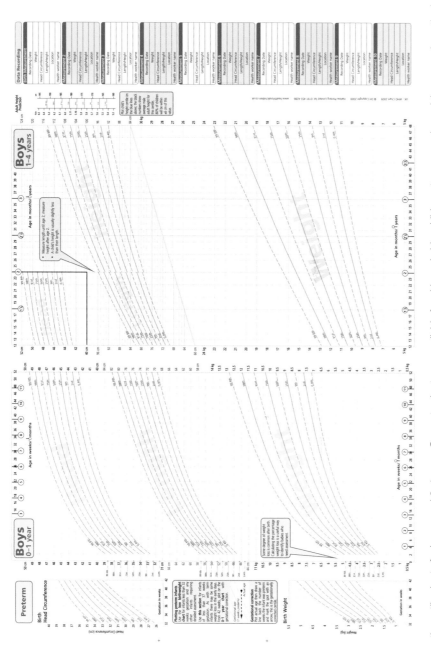

Figure 3.2 Growth centile charts for boys aged 0–4 years. Separate charts are available for girls and older children at www.rcpch.ac.uk/resources/growth-charts. These charts are developed and maintained by RCPCH/WHO/Department of Health. © 2009 Department of Health. Source: RCPCH/WHO/Department of Health. © 2009 Department of Health.

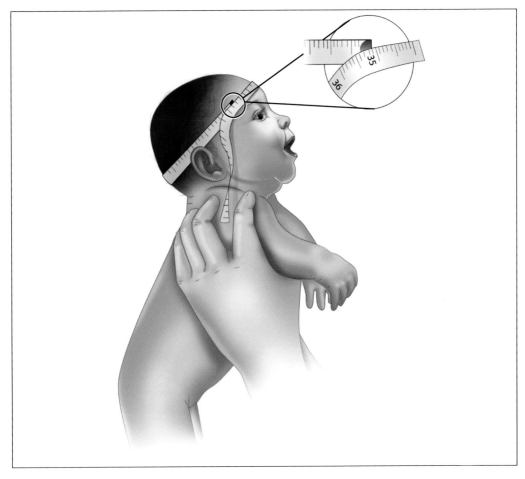

Figure 3.3 Measuring an infant's head circumference: *head circumference* is an important measurement and reflects the volume of the cranial contents with surprising accuracy;

- a good quality, inelastic tape is used;
- the tape passes over the occiput, above the ears, and the prominence of the brow;
- two or three measurements are taken in slightly different planes, and the largest is recorded as the head circumference.

3.2.2 Normal growth

Growth rates are good indicators of general health and nutrition. Children who are growing normally usually have height and weight measurements that progress parallel to the centile lines and are in proportion (i.e. not more than two centile lines difference between height and weight). 95% of healthy children are between the second and ninety-eighth centiles.

3.2.3 Growth velocity and puberty

Growth velocity refers to gain in weight or height over time. Height velocity is measured in cm/year. It is highest in the first year and then gradually falls until the pubertal growth spurt when there is a second smaller peak. Depending on whether puberty starts early or late, a child's height and weight may move away from their 'normal' centile around this time. If puberty is early, growth will accelerate towards a

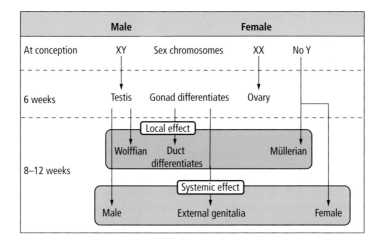

Figure 3.4 Embryonic and fetal sex differentiation.

higher centile and then gradually level off as the rate of the pubertal growth spurt slows. Full assessment of height may require information about pubertal status (Figures 3.5 and 3.6) and bone age (see Section 3.2.5).

3.2.4 Nutritional assessment

Accurate nutritional assessment is difficult and complex. The initial clinical impression is usually valuable. An undernourished child is 'all skin and bone'; the limbs are slender, the bony prominences are conspicuous, and loss of muscle bulk may be observed. In the younger child, this is seen as wasting of the buttocks. Mid-upper arm circumference is measured simply with a tape measure around the arm at the mid-point between the elbow and the shoulder. Centile charts provide reference data but, in the child aged 1–5 years, a circumference less than 14 cm suggests poor nutrition and needs further assessment. If weight loss has been recent, folds of skin on the lower abdomen and inner aspects of the thighs may be seen. Excess fat is most evident on the trunk. Weight for height can be assessed by looking at the relative centiles for the two measurements.

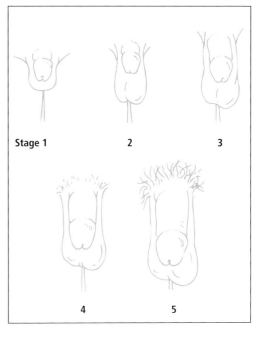

Figure 3.5 Stages of male genital development.
(1) Preadolescent. (2) Enlargement of scrotum and testes.
(3) Increases of breadth of penis and development of glans. (4) Testes continue to enlarge. Scrotum darkens.
(5) Adult: by this time, pubic hair has spread to the medial surface of the thighs.

 PRACTICE POINT

Body mass index (BMI = weight (kg) ÷ height (m)^2) varies with age, and charts are available. A BMI > 20 kg/m^2 in a child of 1–10 years indicates obesity. Calculators are available on the Internet which chart and help to interpret BMI (e.g. go to www.nhs.uk and search 'bmi').

3.2.5 Bone age

Bone age (or skeletal age) is a useful index of growth and maturation. A plain X-ray of the hand and wrist is taken. Calcification of the epiphyses, and later their fusion, is noted for each of the bones around the wrist and compared with standard pictures. The method is complex and requires special skills. In healthy children, bone age relates more closely to height than to age, short children tending to have 'delayed' and tall children 'advanced' bone ages. Significant advance or delay in bone age merits investigation.

3.3 Dental development

Teeth begin to erupt on average in the latter half of the first year, but there is a wide normal range. There are 20 deciduous and 32 permanent teeth; permanent teeth appear from the sixth year. The first molars and central incisors appear first. All teeth have appeared by the age of 14 except the third molars. Teeth appear a few months earlier in girls.

3.4 Sexual development

Human sexual development is concentrated into two brief periods of time: primary sexual development in the embryo (Figure 3.4) and the appearance of secondary sex characteristics during puberty. At puberty, changes occur in response to pituitary gonadotrophins. The trigger for release of these hormones is still unknown. The age of onset of puberty is very variable and is influenced by racial, hereditary and nutritional factors.

In girls in the UK today, breast development begins at 11 years of age on average and pubic hair a little later. Early breast development may be asymmetrical. Mean age of menarche is 13 years, but is commonly between 11 and 15 years. The first signs of puberty are breast development in girls and growth of the testes in boys. In both sexes, puberty is accompanied by an impressive growth spurt, which occurs early in puberty in girls (maximal at age 12 years) and late in puberty in boys (maximal at 14 years) – see Figure 14.5. The progress of puberty is recorded in stages of pubic hair (both sexes), external genitalia (male) and breast development (female) (Figures 3.5 and 3.6). Epiphyseal fusion, with cessation of growth, marks the end of puberty.

3.5 Systems examination

3.5.1 Head and neck

3.5.1.1 Lymph glands

Superficial lymph glands are always palpable in the neck and groins of children. Normal glands are soft, mobile, non-tender and usually not larger than 1–2 cm. Enlarged tonsillar glands, just behind the angle of the jaw, indicate past or present throat infections and may persist for months. Generalized lymphadenopathy suggests systemic illness unless it is due to widespread skin disease (e.g. eczema).

PRACTICE POINT

Benign lymph nodes are smooth, mobile, non-tender, usually not larger than 1–2 cm, may vary in size and persist for many months. Most don't need any investigation. They are common in the neck, less so in the groins and rare in the axillae. Hard, craggy, fixed nodes are unlikely to be benign and need urgent referral.

3.5.1.2 Fontanelles

Anterior fontanelle – is widely open at birth, but varies considerably in size. It closes between 9 and 18 months. Gentle pressure over the fontanelle gives an indication of its tension. The normal fontanelle is relaxed when the infant is resting. It pulsates with the heartbeat. Tension increases when the infant cries or strains.

Changes may provide important clues if supported by other clinical signs:

- Large fontanelle → hydrocephalus
- Small fontanelle → slow brain growth
- Sunken fontanelle → dehydration
- Bulging fontanelle → raised intracranial pressure.

Posterior fontanelle – far back where the sagittal and lambdoid sutures meet. It closes soon after birth.

Third fontanelle – sometimes present in the sagittal suture just in front of the posterior fontanelle. It may be a marker for other congenital abnormality.

3.5.2 Ear, nose and throat

This is an important part of the general examination of any child, especially an ill child. It is difficult in

Breast development

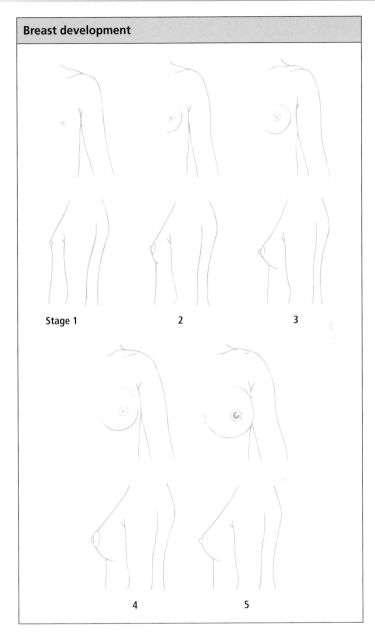

Figure 3.6 Stages of breast development. (1) Preadolescent – elevation of papilla only. (2) Breast bud stage. (3) Further enlargement of breast and areola. (4) Projection of areola and papilla above the level of breast. (5) Mature stage – areola has recessed, papilla projects.

babies, and young children may dislike having their ears examined. Practice makes perfect. Take time to ensure the young child is securely held – this makes for a much easier examination (Figures 3.7 and 3.8).

 OSCE TIP

You will probably not be asked to do ENT examination in a real child in the OSCE, but it is an essential skill in acute paediatrics, and manikins can be used. Make sure you can do it.

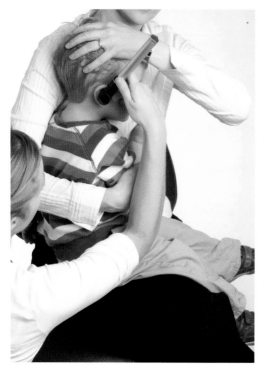

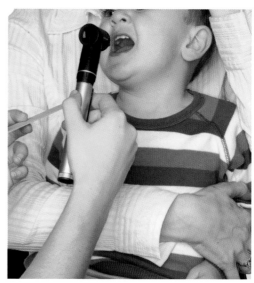

Figure 3.8 Examination of the mouth and throat. Take time to position the child correctly facing towards you on the parent's lap. One of the parent's arms should encircle the child's chest and arms, while the other hand presses on the child's forehead.

Figure 3.7 Ear examination. Examination of the ear is easier and safer if the infant is held correctly. Note the child is held sideways-on against the parent in a firm 'cuddle'. The rear arm should be behind the parent's back. Hold the auroscope between the thumb and index finger, using the remaining fingers to brace against the child's cheek (this protects against damage caused by sudden movement).

3.5.2.1   Ears

- Brace with your fingers against the child's cheek to prevent accidental damage to the meatus with the speculum.
- Draw the pinna gently upwards and backwards to allow a clear view of the eardrums.

3.5.2.2   Nose

Note nasal discharge or bleeding. Although not routine, the nasal mucosa may be examined with the auroscope. Note the colour of the mucosa, the presence of oedema, secretions, polyps or foreign bodies.

3.5.2.3   Mouth and throat

- Note the state of the gums, teeth, tongue and buccal mucosa.

- If children will put their tongue out and say 'ah', the posterior pharynx may be viewed without a tongue depressor. A wooden tongue depressor is well-tolerated by most children. It must be used gently and not placed so far back as to cause gagging. It is difficult to get a good view of the throat in babies.

 PRACTICE POINT

Never examine the throat of a young child with stridor: it may precipitate respiratory obstruction.

3.5.3   Chest and lungs

3.5.3.1   Inspect the chest

- *Hyperinflation* is caused by chronic obstructive airways disease as in bad asthma or seen acutely in conditions such as bronchiolitis.
- *Pectus carinatum*: the sternum is displaced forward, relative to the ribs. Children do not like to hear themselves referred to as pigeon-chested.
- *Pectus excavatum*: a depression in the anterior chest wall above the epigastrium due to a short central tendon of the diaphragm which tethers the lower end of the sternum.

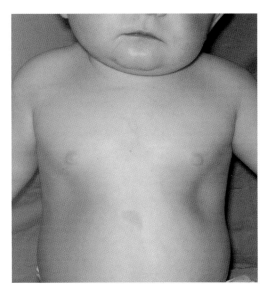

Figure 3.9 Harrison's sulcus. Note the indentation or 'guttering' of the lower ribcage, which is a chronic deformity.

- *Harrison's sulcus.* A bony rib deformity, which is a linear indentation, parallel to and just above the costal margin (Figure 3.9). Its position corresponds to the insertion of the diaphragm and it is due to either increased diaphragmatic pull (chronic respiratory conditions such as poorly controlled asthma) or bone disease such as rickets, where the bones are more easily deformed by normal diaphragmatic action.

> **? OSCE TIP**
>
> In the OSCE, it does not matter if you forget the Latin terms: pectus carinatum is just increased AP diameter with prominent sternum.

3.5.3.2 Assess respiratory effort

- Respiratory rate. Tachypnoea is important. Breathing should be measured at rest over a full 30 s. Normal respiratory rate falls with age: in infants, it should be less than 60/min, and in children, it should be less than 40/min. Rates less than 20 or intermittent apnoea should always raise immediate and urgent concern.
- Pattern of breathing. Prolonged expiration occurs with wheeze. Deep, sighing (acidotic) breathing occurs in diabetic ketoacidosis.

- Recession in the intercostal spaces, epigastrium and suprasternal notch may be seen with increased respiratory effort and obstruction of air flow into the lungs.

> **Signs of respiratory distress**
>
> - Tachypnoea
> - Recession (intercostal, subcostal, suprasternal)
> - Nasal flaring
> - Use of accessory muscles (appears as head bobbing in babies who cannot fix the shoulder girdle)
> - Grunting on expiration (in infants)
> - Cyanosis
> - Difficulty in walking, talking, drinking or speaking.

3.5.3.3 Detect added noises

- Wheeze: a predominantly expiratory sound, due to obstruction in the lower airways. Typical of asthma and bronchiolitis.
- Stridor: a predominantly inspiratory sound, indicating upper airway obstruction and typical of croup or laryngeal oedema.
- Cough: most often arises in the upper respiratory tract. Children tend to swallow sputum rather than spit it out. A barking cough is typical of croup. Paroxysms of coughing with inspiratory 'whoop' occur in whooping cough.

3.5.3.4 Percussion

Place finger firmly, but gently, in contact with the anterior chest wall, and parallel to the ribs. Percuss your own finger lightly. Percuss over the clavicle and the front of the chest and in three positions on each side of the chest posteriorly. In children under 2 years, percussion yields limited information, but is important where auscultation is abnormal or asymmetrical.

3.5.3.5 Auscultation

- Use an appropriately sized stethoscope. An adult-sized stethoscope placed on a newborn baby will pick up heart, breath and bowel sounds all at once! Compare air entry on both sides. In small children, it is normal for breath sounds to be bronchial.
- Coarse crepitations are often transmitted from the throat or upper airways. These may clear if the child coughs first.

PRACTICE POINT **Auscultation**

If a young child finds it hard to take a deep breath, ask them to blow out and listen when they breathe in afterwards.

3.5.3.6 Peak expiratory flow rate (PEFR)

Consider measurement of peak flow in a child old enough to do it (e.g. age 6 years and above). It is interpreted according to height (see Section 20.7.3).

3.5.4 Cardiovascular system

3.5.4.1 Inspection

- Look for increased respiratory rate or other signs of increased work of breathing.
- Watch a baby feeding. The infant sucks well at first, but then has to stop for a rest.

 Poor feeding is a cardinal sign of heart failure.

- Is there cyanosis on rest or on exertion?
- Precordial bulge: the right ventricle pushes the sternum forward.
- Ventricular heave: the right ventricle causes the lower sternum to move forward with each cardiac impulse.

3.5.4.2 Pulse

- The minimum requirement is to count the pulse and to examine its character in both brachials. Check that the femoral pulses are present and that there is no brachio-femoral delay (coarctation of the aorta).
- Rate. Normal rate falls with age.
- Rhythm.
- Character. Small volume in shock; bounding pulse in patent ductus arteriosis.

3.5.4.3 Palpation

- Find the apex beat. It should be in the fourth or fifth intercostal space, just lateral to the nipple
- Check the apex is on the left.
- Thrills are the vibration of a loud murmur. If you do not hear a murmur, you have not felt a thrill.

3.5.4.4 Auscultation

- Listen for two heart sounds.
- Splitting of the second sound is easily heard in children and is usually normal. The gap between the aortic and pulmonary second sounds increases in inspiration.

3.5.4.5 Murmurs

- Timing: pansystolic, ejection systolic, continuous or, rarely, diastolic.
- Quality: describe the sound or character.
- Site of maximum intensity: where?
- Intensity: how loud is it?
- Radiation: can the murmur be heard in the neck or back?

 Intensity grading of heart murmur

1 Barely audible
2 Soft
3 Easy to hear, no thrill
4 Loud, easily audible, thrill
5 Very loud, with easily palpable thrill
6 Audible with the stethoscope held off the chest.

3.5.4.6 Blood pressure

Select an appropriate cuff size (Figure 3.10) – it should be wide enough to cover two-thirds of the distance between the tip of the elbow and shoulder. In practice, this is the largest cuff that will comfortably fit around the upper arm. Too small a cuff yields a falsely high blood pressure. Check the systolic pressure by palpation first, then determine systolic and diastolic pressures by auscultation. Automated methods (e.g. Dinamap) are commonly used in paediatrics. Blood

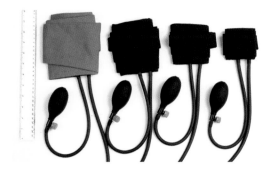

Figure 3.10 Select the correct cuff size for BP measurement.

pressure should be judged against centile charts (search 'BP centiles' at www.nhlbi.nih.gov). In the neonatal period, mean systolic blood pressure is 70 mmHg. From 6 weeks to 10 years of age, mean systolic blood pressure remains around 95 mmHg, and most children will have a systolic blood pressure less than 115 mmHg. Mean systolic blood pressure is 125 mmHg by 16 years of age.

3.5.5 Abdomen and gastrointestinal tract

3.5.5.1 Mouth

The oral cavity should be examined thoroughly. Note cracking and soreness around the lips.

3.5.5.2 Inspection

- Abdominal distension. Normal toddlers are rather pot bellied. The mother will be able to say whether the abdomen is swollen.
- Scars.
- Visible peristalsis.
- Hernia.
- The acutely painful abdomen does not move normally with respiration.

3.5.5.3 Palpation

Is the abdomen soft or tender with guarding? Palpate gently and then more deeply while talking to the child and carefully observing their face for signs of tenderness.

3.5.5.4 Hernia

An umbilical hernia is easily seen (Section 22.2.3.1). Inguinal hernias may not be immediately evident; femoral hernias are hard to find.

3.5.5.5 Hepatomegaly

- The liver is normally palpable 1–2 cm below the costal margin in infants and young children.
- Palpate from the right iliac fossa upwards. The liver edge moves down with respiration.
- Percussion may be helpful.
- The size of the liver is measured below the costal margin in the mid-clavicular line.

3.5.5.6 Splenomegaly

- The spleen tip may be felt in young infants. Palpate from the right iliac fossa, across the abdomen.

- Spleen moves downwards or diagonally on respiration. The notch is palpable. One cannot get above it, and it is felt anteriorly.

3.5.5.7 Renal swelling

- Normal kidneys may be palpable in the newborn period.
- Kidneys felt bimanually.
- Kidneys move down with respiration.

3.5.5.8 Faecal masses

- Frequently felt in the line of the colon and in the left iliac fossa, especially if the child is constipated.

3.5.5.9 Percussion

The liver and large spleen are dull to percussion.

Ascites

- Diffuse swelling, protuberant umbilicus.
- Shifting dullness: gas-filled bowel produces resonant percussion note on the uppermost point of the abdomen. If ascites is present, then when the child lies on his back the abdomen is resonant around the umbilicus and dull in the flanks. Turn the child so that one side is uppermost. The upper flank should now be resonant and the umbilical area dull (Figure 3.11).

3.5.5.10 Auscultation

- Increased bowel sounds: intestinal hurry, e.g. gastroenteritis and early intestinal obstruction.
- Decreased bowel sounds: paralytic ileus.

3.5.5.11 Rectal examination

Rectal examination is rarely indicated in children. It should only be performed by a skilled doctor who can interpret the findings.

Examine stool for colour, consistency and the presence of blood or mucus.

3.5.5.12 Urinalysis

Urine should be examined and tested with a multireagent stick (OSCE station 23.1).

3.5.5.13 Genitalia

Boys

- Is the penis a normal shape? Is the urethral meatus at the tip of the penis or displaced (hypospadias, epispadias)?

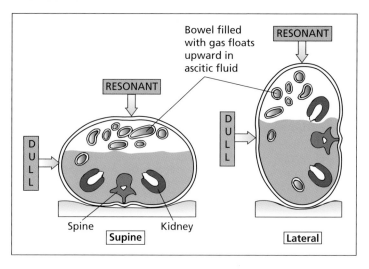

Figure 3.11 Schematic diagram of shifting dullness. Dullness to percussion shifts as the fluid moves and the bowel floats.

- Scrotum and testes. The retractile testis is drawn back up into the scrotum in response to cutaneous stimulation: this is normal in small boys. Gently sweep down the inguinal region (with a warm hand) from lateral to medial to see if you can bring each testis into the scrotum. If the testis cannot be brought into the scrotum, it is undescended or ectopic.
- Scrotal swelling may be fluid (hydrocoele) or hernia. Hydrocoeles transilluminate.

Girls

- Examine vulva and external genitalia.
- Look for soreness, injury, discharge or abnormalities.

3.5.6   Neurology

 PRACTICE POINT

All that is needed is space and time: space for the child to run around and time to watch him (Dr Stuart Green).

3.5.6.1   Motor function

Activity

- Formal examination of tone, power and coordination should be used to help confirm or explain the findings made on simple observation (Table 3.1).
- Does the infant show appropriate head control for age? Is the small child floppy when picked up? Are there symmetry and normal patterns of movement? Can the older child walk or run? Ask the child to sit on the floor and rise quickly (Figure 3.12). Can the child walk on tiptoe or on his heels?
- These observations should be made before reaching for the tendon hammer. Check with the mother first and encourage a child gently. If a child is unable to walk, asking him to do so is not kind.

3.5.6.2   Muscle tone

- The normal infant and young child can touch his ears with his toes. Observe head control and look for hypotonia when the infant is picked up.

Table 3.1 Characteristics of upper and lower motor neurone lesions

	Upper motor neurone	Lower motor neurone
Example	Cerebral palsy	Spina bifida
Strength	Decreased	Decreased
Tone	Increased	Decreased
Reflexes	Increased	Absent/decreased
Clonus	Present	Absent

- Muscle tone is generally assessed on passive movement. Ensure the child is relaxed.
- The most common abnormality of tone is *spasticity* (increased tone around a joint in one direction of movement). The most common groups of muscles affected are the hip adductors (test by abducting the hips) and the plantar flexors (tested by dorsiflexing the foot). When both groups are affected, scissoring and toe pointing are seen.

3.5.6.3   Muscle power

This is best tested in children old enough to cooperate by giving simple commands, e.g. 'squeeze my fingers', 'push me away'. Formal grading of muscle power is seldom used in young children, but the arbitrary

Table 3.2 Grading of muscle power (MRC)

0	No contraction
1	Slight contraction
2	Movement with gravity eliminated
3	Movement against gravity
4	Movement against gravity and resistance
5	Normal power

Source: Adapted from the Medical Research Council Muscle Scale, used with permission.

grades commonly used in adults can be used in older children (Table 3.2). It is best to describe the effects of abnormal power on movement and activity.

3.5.6.4   Muscle wasting

Loss of muscle bulk may be seen in a wide variety of disorders. Hypertrophy of the calf muscles is seen in Duchenne muscular dystrophy (Figure 3.12).

3.5.6.5   Tendon reflexes and clonus

- Reflexes are often easier to elicit in a child than in an adult. The child must be relaxed. Reinforcement may be helpful: ask the child to squeeze his hands together.
- Brisk reflexes in association with spasticity suggest an upper motor neurone (pyramidal) lesion.
- Plantar response may be extensor in the normal child until around the age of walking. In older children, a normal flexor response should be seen.
- *Ankle clonus*, if sustained, is suggestive of an upper motor neurone lesion. It is best tested for with the knee semi-flexed. Dorsiflex the ankle sharply, trying different degrees of pressure. Pressing too lightly or too hard may mask clonus.

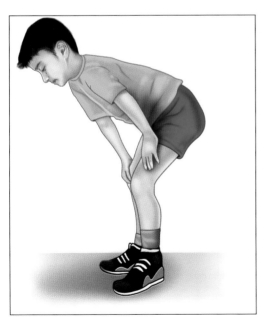

Figure 3.12 Gower's sign. If asked to rise from sitting on the floor, the child turns prone and climbs up his own legs. This indicates limb-girdle weakness and is typical of Duchenne dystrophy.

3.5.6.6   Coordination

This may be tested in children more than 2 years old by the finger–nose and heel–shin manoeuvres. In younger children, it is more helpful to watch for any unsteadiness when playing. A healthy 3-year-old child can stand on one leg briefly and make a good attempt to walk heel-to-toe along a straight line on the floor.

To test for *dysdiadochokinesis*, ask the child to copy you patting the back of one hand as fast as possible and then the other. Even 10-year-olds cannot do it as quickly as an adult can.

3.5.6.7 Sensation and proprioception

A child who has significant abnormalities in this area is likely to show problems when observed in general activities. Full testing of sensation is rarely performed. It is very difficult in infants and toddlers, but enjoyed by older children. Painful stimuli should not be used.

3.5.6.8 Cranial nerves

- Examination often includes inspection of the eyes, external ocular movement and observation for manifest squint (Section 11.4.4).

- Facial nerve function and hearing should be observed. Other tests are only performed if there is indication (Table 3.3).
- Ophthalmoscopy and examination of the fundi are difficult. Looking at the optic disk has been described as 'trying to identify a friend on a passing train'. Ask the child to fix on an object in a dimly lit room, and make sure the ophthalmoscope light is not too bright. Do not worry if you fail – you are in good company!

PRACTICE POINT

To examine the fundi in a young child, ask her to look at an interesting picture, and ask about it while examining. With patience, the disk can often be seen.

- The eye should also be inspected for corneal opacity, abnormality or cataract. If good visualization of the retina is essential in young children, consider referral to the ophthalmologist.

Table 3.3 Tests for cranial nerve function

Nerve	Function	Test
I	Smell	Not often tested
II	Acuity	Simple tests of vision appropriate for age
	Pupils	Direct and consensual light reflex
	Fields	Facing child, who is fixing on your face, test peripheral vision horizontally and vertically
III IV VI	Squint External Ocular movements	See Section 11.4.4 Facing child, watch following of bright object in H pattern. In infants and toddlers, head may be held
V	Motor Masseter Sensation	Clench jaw Light touch on face (avoid corneal reflex)
VII	Facial muscles	Observe smiling or crying. Ask the child to show teeth, close eyes tight and watch eyebrows during upward gaze
VIII	Hearing	8 months: distraction testing. Pre-school: cooperation testing. Over 5 years: audiometry. All ages: tympanometry, auditory evoked responses. Ask parents: is she deaf?
IX X	Swallowing, palate, larynx	Observe swallowing, listen to voice, inspect palatal movement
XI	Trapezius	Ask the child to shrug
XII	Tongue	Ask the child to stick out tongue and move it from side to side

Red reflexes

This describes the reflection of light from the retina, making the pupil appear red (as in the 'red-eye' seen in flash photography). Anything blocking the transmission of light through the eye (e.g. cataract), or changing the colour and character of the retina (e.g. retinoblastoma) will prevent the red reflex. To elicit it, view through the ophthalmoscope in the normal way (focused for infinity), but with the child's face about 0.5–1.0 m away and with the light shining directly at the pupil.

3.5.7 Examination of bones and joints

Fractures are common in childhood and will cause local pain, tenderness and sometimes swelling. Joint disease is not so common, but arthritis and synovitis do occur. Each joint must be examined carefully:

- *Inspection*: Is there swelling or deformity? Does the skin look red? Compare the two sides. Is there wasting of adjacent muscles? If in doubt, measure. If a joint is painful, ask the child to show you how far it will move without pain before you touch it.
- *Palpation*: Does the skin feel hot? Is there tenderness? Is there fluid in the joint? Is there crepitus when the joint moves? Put the joint through the full range of movement in every direction, watching the child's face to be sure you do not hurt him. Compare the two sides.
- *Measurement*: comparison of muscle bulk can be made by measuring the greatest circumference of the calves, upper arm or forearm muscles. Thighs should be measured about their middle, marking the same distance above the patella on the two sides. Leg lengths are measured with the legs in line with the trunk, from the anterior superior iliac spine or the umbilicus to the medial malleolus at the ankle, taking the tape medial to the patella.

3.5.7.1 Joint movements

Joint movement should be tested gently if pain may be present. Active and passive range of movement should be noted. The *hip* movements are internal and external rotation, adduction, abduction, flexion and extension. Hip disease may be associated with buttock wasting and/or leg shortening. All newborns are tested for stability of the hip joint (Section 24.1.7, OSCE station 24.1).

The *knee* normally extends beyond 180° and flexes until the heel touches the buttock. Knee disease is often associated with quadriceps wasting.

The *spine* should be examined for abnormal curvature and for mobility.

 RESOURCE pGALS (Paediatric Gait, Arms, Legs, Spine)

Go to **www.arthritisresearchuk.org** and search for 'pGALS' for videos on how to do a musculoskeletal screening examination in a child, and other useful resources. Download the 'pGALS' app to your phone. See pGALS OSCE Station 3.1 at the end of this chapter for more details.

 # Summary

Examining children is a key skill. You can only learn it by doing it! But we hope this chapter will be a useful starting point, and we encourage you to take every opportunity to hone your skills.

 FOR YOUR LOG

- Make sure you have mastered every system examination adapted for children. Don't forget child development and squints (see Sections 10.2 and 11.4.4).
- Measure child growth (height, weight and head circumference) and be able to plot and interpret a centile chart (including BMI).
- Assessing respiratory distress.
- Know normal and common features, e.g. benign cervical lymph nodes and the normal fontanelle.

 OSCE TIP

- Any systems examination in a child
- Development assessment in a young child.
- Assessment through video of clinical examination findings (e.g. respiratory distress).
- Before a paediatric OSCE, go back to the wards and do a history, a complete examination, and a developmental assessment.

OSCE station 3.1: pGALS examination in a child

Station instructions: 'Please perform a pGALS screen in Ben, who is 9-years-old. Report your findings to the examiner'

Approach: HIGHCOST – introduction, verbal consent, hand hygiene, etc. Ensure child is appropriately clothed, e.g. shorts and t-shirt/vest, bare feet. Child friendly approach throughout with clear explanations/demonstrations and encouraging comments.

Questions
- Any pain or stiffness in joints, muscles or back?
- Any difficulty getting dressed without help? Or lifting something above shoulder level?
- Any problem going up and down steps? Or being able to squat?

Manoeuvres	Suggested commentary (adjust for findings)
Gait and observation	
Observe Ben standing (from front, back and sides)	Ben's posture appears normal, there are no skin rashes, I can see no deformity. In particular, his leg lengths appear equal, I can't see any sign of scoliosis, joint swelling, muscle wasting or flat feet.
Please can you walk across the room, turn round and then come back? Now can you walk on your tiptoes? And now on your heels?	This allows me to assess Ben's feet and ankles, and the joints of the ankles, feet and toes. Ben walks normally. He has normal foot posture and has a good medial longitudinal arch when on tiptoes.
Arms	
Now I want you to copy me: can you hold your hands out straight in front of you?	I can observe good forward flexion of shoulders, and normal elbow, wrist and finger extension.
Can you turn your hands over and make a fist, like this?	Ben has good wrist and elbow supination, and normal flexion of the finger joints.
And can you pinch your index finger and thumb together? (demonstrate) . . . and now touch the tips of each finger with your thumb, like this.	I can see Ben has good manual dexterity and good coordination of the small joints of his fingers.
I'm going to gently squeeze your hand (squeeze the metacarpophalangeal joints).	There is no tenderness in the metacarpophalangeal joints
Next can you put your hands together palm to palms with your elbows horizontal, and now put your hands together back to back, again with your elbows horizontal? (demonstrate)	I can see that Ben has full extension of the small joints of his fingers, and normal wrist extension and flexion, and normal elbow flexion.
Now, please reach up, 'touch the sky', and look at the ceiling.	I observe normal neck extension, shoulder abduction and elbow/wrist extension.
Put your hands behind your neck.	He has normal shoulder abduction, external rotation of his shoulders, elbow flexion
Legs	
Please can you lie on the couch now?	
I'm going to press on your knee (feel for effusion and perform patellar tap).	There is no effusion present at either knee.
Can you bring your heel to your bottom? (each side, one at a time).	Ben has normal knee flexion and extension on active movement.
I'm going to move your leg around with my hand on your knee. (Passive movement: flex knee to 90°, feel for crepitus, flex hip, internally rotate hip.)	Ben has normal passive knee flexion with no crepitus, and normal hip flexion and internal rotation.

Manoeuvres	Suggested commentary (adjust for findings)
Spine (and temporomandibular joint)	
Please can you open your mouth wide and put three fingers in your mouth, like this (demonstrate, fingers vertically aligned).	Ben's temporomandibular joints appear to be normal with no deviation of jaw movement.
Try and touch each shoulder with your ear, like this.	Cervical spine lateral flexion is normal.
And as the last thing, can you bend forward and touch your toes? (Place fingers on spine, observe flexed spine from behind for hump.)	I note he has normal thoracolumbar spine forward flexion and there is no scoliosis.

Concluding: 'Thank you Ben so much for your help. I'm just going to explain to this doctor what I've noticed'.

'In summary, Ben appears to be a healthy 9-year-old boy, and there are no abnormalities on the pGALS screen'.

4

The clinical process

4.1 Investigations and procedures

In general, investigations are more difficult in children, both to carry out and to interpret. Once a decision has been made to take blood, there is a temptation to do more tests than are strictly necessary to spare the child potential distress of another procedure. This should be resisted, because tests done without good reason are rarely helpful and may lead to more unnecessary investigation.

4.1.1 Procedures in children

The power of distraction should not be underestimated, and you can often help with this. This can be as simple as talking, showing interesting toy or game, watching a video and blowing bubbles.

PRACTICE POINT

Reducing procedural discomfort and distress
- parents present
- distraction
- play specialists involved
- topical anaesthetic cream or local anaesthetic
- preparation without misleading (i.e. don't say it's not going to hurt when it will)
- proficient operators with adequate assistance
- getting senior help early if needed

Some procedures routinely require an anaesthetic in young children (e.g. CT head scan, magnetic resonance imaging (MRI) scan), but with preparation and expert input from play specialists this can be avoided, or sometimes sedation is used.

Paediatrics Lecture Notes, Tenth Edition. Jonathan C. Darling and James Yong.
© 2022 John Wiley & Sons Ltd. Published 2022 by John Wiley & Sons Ltd.
Companion website: www.wiley.com/go/lecturenotes/paediatrics10e

Table 4.1 Some investigations that are different in children

Investigation	Difference in children
Full blood count	• higher white cell count in young children • higher haemoglobin at birth, gradually falls to nadir by the second year
Lumbar puncture	• up to 30 lymphocytes allowed in the first month • higher protein level in the first month
ECG	• there is right axis deviation birth, reflecting the relatively bigger right ventricle in foetal life • the axis gradually swings to the left through childhood • for this reason an extra right-sided chest lead (V4R) is included in children • there are many other minor differences that vary with age • be cautious of accepting machine interpretations
CXR	• the thymus may be quite large in small children and appears as a triangular 'sail-like' shape over the right of the mediastinum

4.1.2 Interpreting investigations in children

 Don't assume that because you know what is normal in adults, you can apply the same to children.

The interpretation of many investigations is different in children (see Table 4.1).

4.2 Reaching a diagnosis

> **PRACTICE POINT   Clinical reasoning tools**
>
> • Problem listing/summarising
> • Pattern recognition
> • Probabilistic reasoning
> • Clinical handles
> • Aetiological sieve
> • Rule of parsimony

4.2.1 Problem listing

Begin with a concise problem list summarising all the key clinical features to help you organize your thoughts and apply other tools below. It is helpful to write this at the end of your clinical notes on the history and examination.

4.2.2 Pattern recognition

This is commonly used, especially for common and well-described presentations. The particular cluster of symptom, signs and investigation results follow a recognized pattern described in the textbooks, or (as you gain experience) you have seen before (Table 4.2).

4.2.3 Probabilistic reasoning: clinical handles and likelihood ratios

Logically apply principles of physiology, pathology and aetiology to the clinical presentation, estimating the relative probability of different disease processes being the cause. The probability of a particular disease being the cause of the patient's presentation varies with the presence or absence of different clinical features. Each abnormality (on history, examination or investigation) can be thought of as a clinical 'handle' that allows you to gain some grasp on the problem. Some clinical handles are much more significant than others in making a particular diagnosis likely.

Table 4.2 Pattern recognition

Pattern	Diagnosis
8-month-old with cough, shortness of breath and off feeds, following an upper respiratory infection, has an explosive wet cough, increased respiratory rate, widespread inspiratory crackles and expiratory wheezes in the chest	Bronchiolitis (see Section 20.5.2)
4-month-old with 2 weeks of increasing projectile vomiting, feeding hungrily, blood gas shows hypochloraemic, hypokalaemic, metabolic alkalosis	Pyloric stenosis (see Section 22.2.2.2)
5-year-old with a symmetrical purpuric rash over buttocks, extensor surfaces of legs and arms, abdominal pain, swollen painful ankles, afebrile, full blood count and clotting normal.	IgA vasculitis (Henoch Schonlein Purpura) (see Section 24.3.5)

This corresponds closely to the concept of 'Likelihood Ratios' with regard to clinical investigations. When you are considering a diagnosis in a patient, there is a 'prior probability' of the disease being present (for example, the prior probability of bacterial sepsis in a child presenting to the A&E with a fever of 38 °C is low). A test with a high likelihood ratio increases that probability much more than one with a low likelihood ratio. This means it helps you rule out or rule in a diagnosis.

If we could do an immediate PCR (polymerase chain reaction test) for a panel of bacteria that cause sepsis in children, and it was positive, we would be now be very worried about bacterial sepsis – the positive test has changed a low prior probability into a high 'post-test probability'. Similarly, a negative PCR would be reassuring and make such a diagnosis lower than the prior probability. This test would therefore have a high likelihood ratio, because it has a big impact on the diagnostic probability of sepsis.

Unfortunately, such a test is not yet commonly available immediately, and we use proxy indicators such as blood CRP and white count, which have much lower likelihood ratios for any given level (but are still useful). Likelihood ratios can be calculated precisely from studies of how tests perform in different populations and are based on sensitivity and specificity.

In practice, most clinicians don't use precise numerical figures for likelihood ratios of the tests they are requesting, but these concepts underpin clinical reasoning, even if not explicitly described in clinical notes. Doctors build up a 'feel' for characteristics of the tests they use, through medical education, evidence and clinical practice. Wherever possible, review the data for tests you use.

Each positive or negative clinical finding (whether in the history, examination or investigation phase) can be thought of as a 'test' with its own test characteristics and likelihood ratio. Through clinical reasoning, we amalgamate all this clinical information and (in effect) estimate how much the prior probability of different diseases under consideration has been changed upwards or downwards. We recognize that in this process, some clinical findings and some test findings are more useful than others: they can be thought of as being strong or weak clinical handles (Table 4.3), or having high or low likelihood ratios.

Strong and weak clinical handles

Strong handles have a large impact on the likelihood of a particular diagnosis

Weak handles have little impact on the likelihood of a particular diagnosis (Table 4.3)

4.2.4 Red flags

🔑 Red flags are warning features that are ignored at your peril! For example, bile-stained vomiting means bowel obstruction until proved otherwise.

As part of your paediatric placement, and from this text, you will start to build a feel for what are strong and weak clinical handles, and what are red flags. Use these to help with your diagnostic reasoning.

Table 4.3 Strong and weak 'handles' for diagnosis

Strength	Feature	Diagnosis being considered	Comment	Likelihood ratio
Strong	Bilateral proptosis	Graves disease	Presence is pathognomic (its presence makes that diagnosis virtually certain)	High
Weak	Moderate cervical lymphadenopathy (e.g. eight smooth mobile nodes of about 1–2 cm in diameter) Non-specific erythematous rash on the trunk	Kawasaki disease	Both these signs are common and have many causes both singly and even in combination. Their presence has limited diagnostic value.	Low

their are signs of life which include movement, normal breathing or coughing.

Give 15 compressions and then two breaths and continue with this pattern with minimum interruption.

 PRACTICE POINTS

The aim of cardiac massage is to compress the heart, ejecting its contents. Compression should be provided over the lower half of the sternum. The aim is to compress the chest one-third of its depth at a rate of around 100-120/min. Release pressure between compressions to allow complete chest recoil.

5.1.3.1 Child (Figure 5.4)

The heel of the hand is placed over the lower half of the sternum. In bigger children, both hands may be used as in adults.

5.1.3.2 Infant (Figure 5.5)

If you are on your own, two fingers are placed over the lower half of the sternum to provide compressions. If

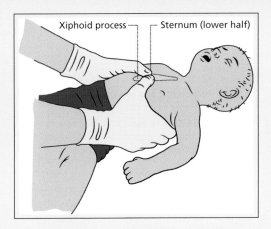

Figure 5.5 Chest compression for an infant. *Source:* Ian K. Maconochie, Robert Bingham, Christoph Eich, Jesús López- Herce, Antonio Rodríguez-Núñez, Thomas Rajka, Patrick Van de Voorde, David A. Zideman, Dominique Biarent, Koenraad G. Monsieurs, Jerry P. Nolan, "European Resuscitation Council Guidelines for Resuscitation 2015 Section 6. Paediatric life support", Resuscitation, 2015, © Elsevier.

there is more than one person, use both hands. The two thumbs are placed in the lower sternum pointing towards the infant's head. The fingers of the hands encircle the chest.

If you are on your own and have a phone available, call for help immediately after the rescue breaths and while proceeding to the next step. If no phone or help is available, give 1 min of CPR and then go for help.

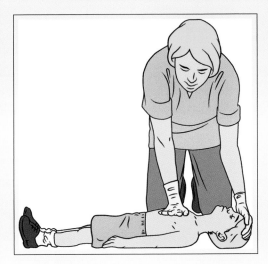

Figure 5.4 Chest compression with one hand. *Source:* Ian K. Maconochie, Robert Bingham, Christoph Eich, Jesús López- Herce, Antonio Rodríguez-Núñez, Thomas Rajka, Patrick Van de Voorde, David A. Zideman, Dominique Biarent, Koenraad G. Monsieurs, Jerry P. Nolan, "European Resuscitation Council Guidelines for Resuscitation 2015 Section 6. Paediatric life support", Resuscitation, 2015, © Elsevier.

5.2 Recognition of impending or imminent collapse

There are two main mechanisms of collapse in children and infants. These are respiratory failure and shock. Each has many causes. Early recognition of a child's worsening condition will allow the team to intervene before collapse occurs. The younger the child, the more quickly he will deteriorate. It can be very difficult to predict these problems in young infants.

This section describes the progress from respiratory distress to failure and the evolution of shock. In many conditions, both occur together.

5.2.1 Respiratory distress and failure

 Respiratory distress is common – it means increased work of breathing.

Respiratory failure is uncommon – it means that the child's breathing is insufficient to ensure adequate oxygenation and ventilation.

 PRACTICE POINTS
Signs of respiratory distress

- Increased respiratory rate
- Intercostal or subcostal recession, tracheal tug and nasal flaring
- Use of accessory muscles and head-bobbing
- Grunting

 Remember that in neuromuscular disease, central respiratory depression or exhaustion, the signs of respiratory distress may be reduced or absent.

PRACTICE POINTS
Signs of respiratory failure

The following raise concern that respiratory distress is leading to respiratory failure. Here, the child or infant's breathing is not enough to ensure oxygenation and the removal of carbon dioxide. Any of the following should raise concern:

- The respiratory rate is very rapid, irregular or is becoming slow in the absence of recovery
- Cyanosis
- Poor oxygen saturation readings
- Poor response to facial oxygen
- Increasing tachycardia or bradycardia
- Apnoea or respiratory arrest
- Altered level of consciousness (agitation or decreased consciousness).

This list provides the features of respiratory failure. Those lower on the list mark a more severe and worrying picture.

In the presence of respiratory distress, a child should be monitored carefully and given oxygen. Full clinical assessment (history, examination and investigations) will provide a diagnosis and guide specific treatment (e.g. antibiotics for pneumonia).

If there is known or suspected respiratory failure, it is essential to seek urgent help. Do the following:

- Support, comfort and assess
- Ensure there is a patent airway
- Give oxygen
- Consider oxygen saturation monitoring, titrate oxygen saturations to 94-98%, and seek help.

The child should be transferred to a place that can provide high dependency or intensive care.

5.2.2 Shock

The word shock is used widely. In some medical use, it refers to extreme illness often requiring full intensive care. Circulatory shock may progress to this stage but also means the situation where the child is poorly perfused and where there is danger of progression to life-threatening or damaging circulatory failure or even arrest.

 Shock occurs when the circulation is not adequate to maintain organ perfusion.

Shock is common particularly in young children and infants. The most common reason is hypovolaemia due to dehydration. Any other cause of loss of circulating volume will lead to shock. This may include blood loss or sepsis (when fluids leak out of the vascular space). Occasionally, there is a primary cardiac problem so that the heart is not pumping adequately. The diagnosis of shock depends upon clinical examination.

PRACTICE POINTS
Features indicating shock

- Poor peripheral circulation with cool hands and feet
- Prolonged capillary refill time (>2 s) (Section 3.1.6)
- Increased heart rate
- Weak or thready peripheral pulses
- Direct evidence of poor organ perfusion (poor urine output, metabolic acidosis)
- Decreased blood pressure
- Altered level of consciousness.

worsening severity

As the cause of shock, e.g. dehydration (hypovolaemia), worsens, the child will initially show compensation. The compensatory features include the rising pulse and diminished perfusion of the peripheries. Intervention at this stage is highly successful. A child will maintain normal blood pressure by these compensatory methods until decompensation begins to occur. This is followed rapidly by life-threatening deterioration.

Recognition of compensated shock or early signs of decompensation is vitally important. The administration of volume to an infant with dehydration or hypovolaemia of any cause is life saving. Give intravenous fluid boluses of 10ml/kg of crystalloids for treatment of shock. Response to the bolus should be reassessed and repeated if required.

PRACTICE POINTS

So much of acute paediatric care and resuscitation is helped by knowing a child's weight. It would be ideal to get the actual weight of the child, but in an emergency situation this may not be possible. There are different ways of estimating body weight such as the use of centile charts and formulas. One commonly used formula for children aged between 1 and 10 years, Weight = 2(Age in years + 4), is approximate but useful.

5.3 Paediatric advanced life support

If you pursue a career looking after children, you will need to learn these skills and remain updated. There are four main areas:

- Management of the airway
- Vascular access
- Drugs
- Management of cardiopulmonary arrest.

5.3.1 Airway management

Support and maintenance of the airway is a key clinical skill. The simplest and most important aspect is position. In children, an oral airway may be used if the tongue is obstructing ventilation in the child with diminished conscious level. The correct size of oral airway is inserted gently under direct vision using a tongue depressor and torch or the laryngoscope.

If a child is not breathing, ventilations can usually be achieved with a bag and mask. Mask ventilation is important at all ages but it is a skill that must be learned by practical instruction.

An airway may be achieved with a laryngeal mask or tracheal intubation. These specialist techniques require the selection of the correct equipment, specific training and continuing practice.

5.3.2 Vascular access

PRACTICE POINTS

In an emergency, this is achieved with:
- Peripheral intravenous line (usually limiting yourself to 2–3 attempts).
- Intraosseous access – used in life-threatening situations in the unconscious child. If peripheral access cannot be obtained, a specially designed needle is inserted into the proximal tibia avoiding the growth plates. Samples may be taken for investigations. Fluids and drugs may be given through the line.

5.3.3 Drugs

A number of drugs are used during resuscitation. The two most commonly used are oxygen and adrenaline.

Oxygen should be given to any infant or child who has collapsed or who is in danger of collapse. It is given to the child in respiratory distress during assessment. Oxygen may be given by face mask or used with bag/mask ventilation or tracheal intubation.

TREATMENT   Adrenaline

- Catecholamine (alpha and beta stimulant)
- Vasoconstriction
- Raises blood pressure
- Increased myocardial contractility
- Cardiac arrest

Adrenaline is also called epinephrine.

Adrenaline may be given intravenously or through an intraosseous line. It can be given through the endotracheal tube. It is also helpful in the management of anaphylaxis (acute allergic collapse).

TREATMENT

Adrenaline is a dose that all doctors in paediatrics should know: 10 micrograms/kg (0.1 mL/kg of 1 : 10 000) initial dose

5.3.4   Cardiopulmonary arrest

The initial management of cardiopulmonary arrest is as described for BLS.

PRACTICE POINTS

If there is no cardiac output, the problem falls into one of two groups:

• Asystole or pulseless electrical activity. The heart has stopped or is showing electrical activity without contractions. This will not respond to an electric shock. The airway is secured, the child is ventilated, and cardiopulmonary resuscitation and adrenaline are given. Any cause is treated.

• Ventricular fibrillation or pulseless ventricular tachycardia. These conditions are shockable. Defibrillation is used, and other drugs may be helpful.

5.3.5   Foreign body airway obstruction (FBAO)

Choking with airway obstruction is not uncommon in young children. Death is rare. Simple measures are very effective. Most children who choke do so whilst they are playing or eating. The result is that most episodes are observed, and intervention is successful, whilst the child is still conscious.

First assess whether the child has an effective cough or not (Figure 5.6). If the child is able to cough and respond, simply encourage them to do so and continue to assess. If you have any concerns, seek help.

If coughing is becoming ineffective, call for help immediately and perform one of the procedures that give an artificial cough. The artificial cough in the conscious child is provided by back blows or abdominal/chest thrusts.

PRACTICE POINTS
General signs of FBAO

• Witnessed episode
• Coughing/choking
• Sudden onset
• Recent history of playing with/eating small objects

Obstructed airway	Airway clear
Unable to vocalize	Crying or verbal response
Quiet or silent cough	Loud cough
Unable to breathe	Able to take a breath
Cyanosis	Pink
Decreased consciousness	Fully responsive

To give back blows, it is best to have the child head downwards and in a prone position with the lower jaw supported to open the airway. The infant can be picked up. A small child can be placed across the lap, whilst older children will need to be supported.

Five back blows are given. The heel of the hand is used to provide a firm blow between the shoulder blades. They work best if the child is head down because the manoeuvre is then assisted by gravity.

Chest thrusts are used in children under 1 year of age. These are like cardiac compressions but sharper and given at a slower rate. Five chest thrusts are given. Abdominal thrusts are used in children over 1 year. This is the Heimlich manoeuvre. Your clenched fist is placed between the umbilicus and the xiphisternum whilst standing behind the child. The other hand grasps the fist. A sharp upwards pull is given.

Once the airway obstruction is relieved, a child will usually recover if they are conscious at the time.

If the child becomes unconscious, place him supine. Examine the mouth. If there is a foreign body visible, then remove it. Do not simply place a finger in the mouth in the hope of finding something. Give mouth-to-mouth resuscitation. After five breaths, give cardiac compressions. Repeat artificial respiration, again examining the mouth for the presence of a foreign body which has become dislodged.

Genetics

Chapter map

Childhood and foetal life is when many genetic problems present. It is important to understand the principles of inheritance and the wide variety of genetic disease. The clinician needs to know about the range of investigations in suspected genetic disease and have an approach to genetic counselling. This chapter does not deal with the individual conditions, many of which can be found elsewhere in this book.

6.1   The human genome

Successful sequencing of the genome was announced on 26 June 2000. Understanding of structure has preceded explanation of function. Current knowledge offers a wealth of new diagnostic tests, increasing therapeutic benefits and the future possibility of gene therapy.

The diploid human cell contains DNA extending to around six billion base pairs in 23 chromosome pairs. Only 2% of DNA codes for protein expression in some 20 000 genes. Some of the remaining DNA offers regulation and control of gene expression, genetic replication and chromosomal architecture, while the function of other non-coding DNA is not yet known.

The base-pair structure of DNA allows replication. During cell division, chromosomes align, replicate and divide. In *mitosis*, identical diploid daughter cells result. In *meiosis*, haploid gametes are produced: eggs and sperm containing half the genetic material, with just one of each of the pairs of chromosomes. In meiosis, genetic material may be swapped between chromosomes, while all cell division carries potential for mutation.

Genes code for polypeptide sequences and these may constitute or may be built into proteins. Post-translational changes modify structure and function and result in functional proteins.

Paediatrics Lecture Notes, Tenth Edition. Jonathan C. Darling and James Yong.
© 2022 John Wiley & Sons Ltd. Published 2022 by John Wiley & Sons Ltd.
Companion website: www.wiley.com/go/lecturenotes/paediatrics10e

'It has not escaped our notice that the specific pairing we have postulated immediately suggests a possible copying mechanism for the genetic material'. Watson, J.D. and Crick, F.H.C. (1953) Molecular structure of nucleic acids: a structure for deoxyribose nucleic acid. *Nature*, 4356, 25 April, 171: 737–8; see also Figure 6.1.

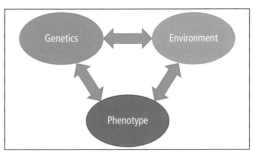

Figure 6.2 There is a complex interaction between genotype, environment and phenotype.

 RESOURCE

Useful refresher videos and animations on DNA and the human genome can be found at:
- **www.biointeractive.org** (search for 'DNA')
- **www.dnalc.org/resources**
- **www.dnatube.com** (e.g. search 'DNA' or 'DNA transcription')

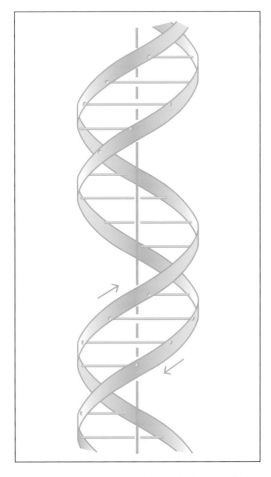

Figure 6.1 DNA – the Nobel Prize winning description of the double helix. *Source:* Watson and Crick (1953).

The potential for errors is massive, but most do not result in disease. It is important to understand the principles underlying genetic disease for diagnosis, prognosis, treatment and genetic counselling.

For any characteristic (height, blood pressure, etc.), our phenotype (the way we are) is the result of complex interaction between our genotype (genetic material related to that characteristic) and our environment (Figure 6.2).

6.2 Genetic mechanisms of disease

- Chromosomal
  - Abnormal number (aneuploidy)
  - Translocation (balanced or unbalanced)
  - Duplication
  - Deletion
  - Copy number variation (abnormal numbers of copies of section of DNA)
- Single gene disorders
  - Mutations
    - Missense (protein product is abnormal, e.g. amino acid substitution)
    - Nonsense (protein product is not complete)
    - Triplet repeat (base-pair triplets)
- Gene imprinting (e.g. modification of gene expression by gender of parent)
- Mitochondrial DNA abnormalities
- Multifactorial inheritance

6.2.1 Chromosomal abnormalities

Aneuploidy means that there is an extra chromosome (e.g. Trisomy 21, Down syndrome; 47XXY, Klinefelter syndrome) or one missing (e.g. 45XO, Turner syndrome). Most aneuploidy arises because of non-disjunction (failure of the pair of chromosomes to separate), and often, it results in spontaneous miscarriage. Down syndrome (trisomy 21), Edward syndrome (trisomy 18), Patau syndrome (trisomy 13) and the sex chromosome aneuploidies account for most infants with abnormal chromosome number. Risk of Down syndrome aneuploidy rises with maternal age.

> Down syndrome is most commonly due to non-disjunction. In around 5% of affected children, other patterns are seen: unbalanced translocation (see Figure 6.3) and mosaicism (the phenotype varies with the balance in number between two cell lines, one of which is trisomy 21).

Translocations occur when a part of one chromosome is stuck to another. If the total chromosome content is normal or near normal (a balanced translocation), the phenotype may be normal. The risk for this person is that their offspring may inherit an unbalanced karyotype.

The other chromosomal abnormalities are associated with a wide variety of phenotypes. Some deletions or duplications may be a chance finding in a healthy child or their family. On the other hand, some are small and not visible on microscopy, yet may result in a variety of important syndromic abnormalities (e.g. 22q deletions: Di George syndrome spectrum with hypocalcaemia, T-cell deficiency, cardiac defects).

> 🔑 A syndrome is a phenotype with a recognizable pattern of various abnormalities or problems.

6.2.2 Single gene disorders

These may adopt the classical Mendelian patterns of inheritance.

Symbols for a genetic pedigree are shown in Figure 6.4.

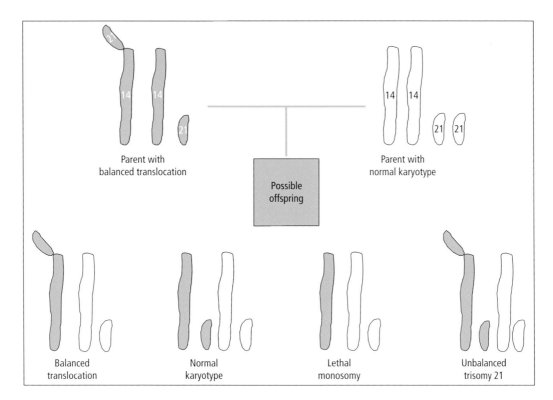

Figure 6.3 A balanced 21 translocation in a healthy parent can result in Down syndrome in the child.

The features of each pattern in a family are described below. You do not need to learn lists of inheritance patterns but should know some of the commoner ones.

Discussion of individual conditions here is to illustrate patterns of inheritance. Please see other chapters for discussion of conditions that are more common or important in paediatrics.

> One phenotype may be the result of a number of different mutations.
> The phenotype may vary between family members who share a genetic abnormality, reflecting variation in expression and penetrance.

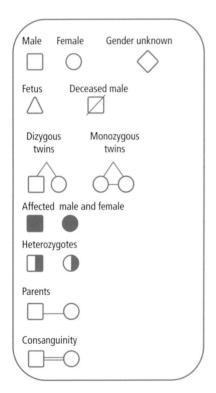

Figure 6.4 Symbols for genetic pedigree.

6.2.2.1 Autosomal dominant (Figure 6.5)

- Parents affected
- Females and males affected
- Female and male transmission
- 50% recurrence risk
- High new mutation rates
- Variable penetrance in some conditions

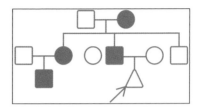

Figure 6.5 Autosomal dominant: parents seek advice on the risk to the foetus

Autosomal dominant conditions

- Achondroplasia
- Huntington's chorea
- Polyposis coli
- Marfan syndrome
- Tuberous sclerosis
- Myotonic dystrophy
- von Willebrand disease

 Trinucleotide repeat disorders

- Trinucleotide repeats (triplet repeat) are normal up to a certain number in some genes. The area is unstable, may expand on the transmission to the next generation and cause disease.
- Anticipation is seen – earlier presentation and greater severity with successive generations.
- Most are autosomal dominant (e.g. myotonic dystrophy – chromosome 19).
- Fragile X is X-linked recessive (see below).

In some dominant conditions, phenotype varies even in the same family. In achondroplasia, the new mutation rate is 50%. Huntingdon's chorea and polyposis do not present until after childhood.

6.2.2.2 Autosomal recessive (Figure 6.6)

- Parents not affected
- Parents heterozygote carriers
- 1 in 4 risk of condition if carrier parents
- 2 in 3 risk of unaffected sibling being carrier
- More common with consanguinity (Section 1.3.3)

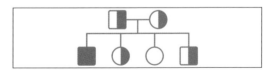

Figure 6.6 Cystic fibrosis: a 1 in 4 risk of affected offspring.

Autosomal recessive conditions

- Cystic fibrosis
- Phenylketonuria
- Sickle cell disease
- Thalassaemia
- Various inborn errors of metabolism (e.g. congenital adrenal hyperplasia)

Rates of gene carriage vary greatly between ethnic groups (e.g. cystic fibrosis carriage in Europe is around 1 in 25, while considerably lower across Asia). Most parents will not know that they carry the rare gene until they have a child with another carrier.

6.2.2.3   X-linked recessive (Figure 6.7)

- Affects males
- Carrier female usually unaffected
- 50% of boys of carrier mother affected
- 50% of daughters of carrier mother are carriers
- 100% of daughters of affected men are carriers
- No transmission from father to son
- New mutations not uncommon

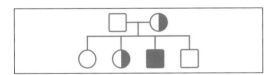

Figure 6.7 Haemophilia A: there is a 1 in 2 chance that girls will be carriers and boys will be affected.

X-linked recessive conditions

- Fragile X
- Duchenne muscular dystrophy
- Haemophilia A and B
- G6PD deficiency
- Red-green colour blindness

The abnormality on one X chromosome is not usually sufficient to lead to disease in the carrier woman. In some women, the Lyon phenomenon (random inactivation of one of the X chromosomes) may result in disease. In fragile X (an important cause of language and developmental problems), women may have mild learning difficulties (Section 11.3.2).

6.2.3   Gene imprinting

Certain genes express differently depending on whether they are inherited from the mother or the father. Current understanding suggests that this is rare in clinical disease.

Affected individuals have the unopposed effect of maternally or paternally inherited genes. This occurs because of a mutation in the gene on one chromosome or because of inheritance of two copies of the gene from the same parent (uniparental disomy).

Example of imprinting (part of chromosome 15q)

Two different disorders result (both rare), depending on whether the maternal or paternal contribution of this imprinted gene is lacking:

- No *paternal* contribution
  - Mutation of the paternally inherited gene, *or*
  - Maternal uniparental disomy
- *Prader–Willi syndrome* (short stature, obesity, eating and behaviour problems, hypogonadism)

- No *maternal* contribution
  - Mutation of the maternally inherited gene, *or*
  - Paternal uniparental disomy
- *Angelman's syndrome* (ataxia, motor problems, abnormal behaviour apparently happy, epilepsy)

6.2.4   Mitochondrial DNA abnormalities

- Maternal inheritance (mitochondria are acquired in the cytosol of the ovum)
- Rare conditions affecting tissues with high energy needs
- Tissues affected: eyes, brain, liver, muscle

6.2.5   Polygenic or multifactorial conditions

The characteristics of our phenotypes have many origins. Some are genetic. Growth has genetic and environmental drivers. Complex features like intelligence are clearly multifactorial.

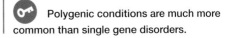 Polygenic conditions are much more common than single gene disorders.

Patterns of inheritance are not well defined, and calculation of risk for polygenic disease is based upon studies of populations. If a family has such a condition (e.g. atopy, diabetes), risk increases with the number of close relatives who are affected.

It is increasingly evident that the health of the foetus and young child has long-term implications for adult health. *Programming* refers to the ability of the early environment during a critical period of development to influence long-term outcome (e.g. the small foetus is more likely to suffer coronary artery disease or diabetes at the age of 60 years).

This makes foetal and childhood well-being the birthplace of adult health.

 Polygenic or multifactorial conditions

- Atopy (e.g. asthma, eczema)
- Spina bifida
- Cleft lip and palate
- Congenital heart disease
- Adult coronary heart disease
- Adult hypertension
- Diabetes
- Epilepsy

6.3 Investigations

6.3.1 Karyotype

Chromosomes are separated during cell division, allowing counting and examination for defects (Figure 11.1). Banding studies (staining) allow definition of chromosomes or parts of chromosomes in duplication or deletion. Resolution is limited by microscopy.

6.3.2 FISH (fluorescence in situ hybridisation)

A fluorescent labelled specific DNA probe sequence binds to complementary DNA on the chromosome. The probe can be seen because it is fluorescent. This can be used to count chromosomes without waiting for a full karyotype. Searching for part of chromosome 21 will show three areas of fluorescence in Down syndrome. Fluorescence in situ hybridisation (FISH) can also look for specific genes or abnormalities or localize a known DNA sequence.

6.3.3 DNA analysis

Specific gene probes are increasingly available. Clearly, they require that the practitioner suspects the condition being tested for.

DNA microarray comprises multiple DNA probes applied simultaneously. This allows more rapid and accurate detection of a wide variety of abnormalities and the search for duplications and deletions.

Polymerase chain reaction (PCR) uses a DNA replication enzyme to achieve exponential increases in the number of copies of a specific section of DNA. PCR amplification makes it much easier to study the DNA. PCR is used to detect small amounts of specific DNA (e.g. detection of Herpes virus in CSF).

6.3.4 Array CGH (comparative genomic hybridisation)

This screens the whole genome to detect changes in copy number of genetic material (such as duplications or deletions) compared to a 'reference' genome. It searches for abnormalities across thousands of loci all at once, compared to FISH which is targeted at specific loci. It may be used for children with unexplained learning difficulties or developmental delay and where there are multiple congenital abnormalities.

6.3.5 Next-generation sequencing

The original technology for genome sequencing was slow and laborious, taking over a decade to produce a first draft of the human genome. It is being superseded by techniques which sequence millions of DNA fragments in parallel and then piece them all together by mapping to a reference genome. This means that a whole genome can be sequenced in a matter of hours. This is generally still a research tool, but will likely become part of routine clinical testing over time.

 Research Trail
The 100 000 genomes project

This is an NHS Project to sequence 100 000 genomes of patients affected by rare diseases or cancer. These data are combined with medical records to produce a research resource to transform our understanding and treatment of disease.

Next Research Trail on page 74

6.4 Approach to suspected genetic disease

PRACTICE POINT

Constant vigilance is necessary to detect inherited disease.

Benefits of early diagnosis of genetic disease

- Families are often helped by having a diagnosis
- Prognosis
- Early intervention during or before disease
- Genetic counselling

It is important to approach a potential genetic diagnosis with some caution. Accuracy is key, usually demanding a multiprofessional team including Clinical Genetics. The implications for the child and her family may be massive. Premature mention of a possible genetic diagnosis may lead a family to deep and unnecessary anxiety – access to detailed and full, and occasionally inaccurate, information is easy for anyone who can find Google.

RESOURCE

The Online Mendelian Inheritance in Man database (OMIM) at **www.ncbi.nlm.nih.gov/omim** is a useful compendium of human genes and genetic phenotypes.

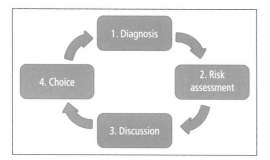

Figure 6.8 Genetic counselling – key steps.

6.4.1 Genetic counselling (Figure 6.8)

An accurate diagnosis is ideal for all. Not uncommonly, a firm diagnosis may be difficult, and often, syndromic diagnoses are made on probability rather than certainty.

Risks for the child and family require careful and complex assessment. Many genetic conditions vary greatly in how much they affect individuals even within one family. Naturally, families will be drawn to expect the same problems with the same diagnosis. The number and gravity of possible outcomes in some conditions (e.g. neurofibromatosis) can be bewildering and cause great worry.

Complex issues in genetic counselling

- Recurrence risk in a family
- Carrier detection in healthy parents, siblings and extended family
- Paternity
- Predictive testing of children who may be presymptomatic
- Reproductive choices including foetal intervention

The complexity and ethical difficulties that arise in this area of medicine are many. Families may seek testing for a genetic disorder in the hope of a reassuring result. This should not take place without careful counselling about the implications of an abnormal test result. Testing of children for diseases that will only affect them as adults and where early intervention does not bring clear benefit (e.g. Huntingdon's chorea, adult polycystic kidney disease) is not generally accepted.

PRACTICE POINT

Clinical Genetics services have great expertise in this area and work closely with paediatrics.

A careful, clear and honest explanation of these complex issues to a concerned family is very challenging. Often families will need to be seen on a number of occasions.

 Good information given with care and compassion will enable families to make the right choices.

Summary

You should now understand the main mechanisms of inherited disease, the variety of patterns of inheritance and something of the clinical approach to investigation, diagnosis and counselling. The immediately obvious complexity is the reason why the child and family are usually best helped by a combined team of paediatrics, community services and clinical genetics.

 FOR YOUR LOG

- Include a family tree in your paediatric histories and extend when concerned about inherited disorders.
- Be able to recognize different genetic mechanisms of inheritance.
- If there is an opportunity during paediatrics, or elsewhere in your course, observe genetic counselling.

 OSCE TIP

- Questions about a pedigree.
- Counselling about simple problems related to inherited or multifactorial conditions.

SBAs

Q6.1 You are asked to counsel a family who have a child with cystic fibrosis. They are planning to have another child and want to know the risk of this child being affected and the risk that the child may be a carrier for cystic fibrosis.

Which of the following would be the appropriate advice?

a. Risk of having CF 1 in 2; Risk of being a carrier 1 in 4
b. Risk of having CF 1 in 2; Risk of being a carrier 2 in 3
c. Risk of having CF 1 in 3; Risk of being a carrier 1 in 4
d. Risk of having CF 1 in 4; Risk of being a carrier 1 in 2
e. Risk of having CF 1 in 4; Risk of being a carrier 2 in 3

Q6.2 You are reviewing a 14-year-old girl in clinic because of delayed puberty. They have never had a period, and they report that there is no breast development, and no pubic or axillary hair. Their height is on the 0.4th centile.

What is the most appropriate initial genetic investigation?

a. CGH array
b. DNA analysis
c. FISH
d. Karyotype
e. Next-generation sequencing

For SBA answers, see page 366.

Foetal medicine

Chapter map

Multidisciplinary collaboration is the key to foetal medicine. Good contraceptive advice is important for the young person, while assisted conception allows more couples the joy of parenthood. Primarily an obstetric specialty, advice to the expectant couple often provides diagnostic and ethical problems, demanding input from paediatrics, genetics and surgery. You should understand that ultrasound, amniocentesis, chorionic villus sampling, foetal blood sampling, DNA analysis and fetoscopy allow assessment of foetal health, early detection of many anomalies and sometimes treatment of the foetus, taking Down syndrome and spina bifida as important examples.

7.1   Control of fertility

7.1.1   Contraception

In developing countries, high birth rates and high child mortality tend to go hand in hand. Medical care reduces mortality from disease, but large family size threatens good nutrition, education and socioeconomic growth. Safe, effective, cheap contraception coupled with education is key.

In Europe, the challenge of providing good, supportive advice to teenagers is widely acknowledged. The UK is now seeing a fall in the teenage pregnancy rate, which in 2016 was around 19/1000 15- to 17-year-olds.

PRACTICE POINT

Gillick competency: This important ethical concept arose when the courts decided that a teenager could obtain contraception without parental knowledge. The principle is that a competent teenager may seek treatment or advice as long as the treating doctor is convinced that the child understands the implications of their choice.

7.2   Antenatal and pre-pregnancy care

Preparation for a baby is aided by good physical and emotional health in both parents. Hereditary conditions should be discussed.

Paediatrics Lecture Notes, Tenth Edition. Jonathan C. Darling and James Yong.
© 2022 John Wiley & Sons Ltd. Published 2022 by John Wiley & Sons Ltd.
Companion website: www.wiley.com/go/lecturenotes/paediatrics10e

PRACTICE POINT

Women should be immunized against rubella before conception. All but the most essential drugs should be stopped before pregnancy. Smoking and alcohol should be avoided.

Some social and behavioural factors increase risk of problems:

- Socioeconomic deprivation: ↑ low birthweight; ↑ prematurity; ↑ perinatal mortality
- Young mothers: ↑ foetal growth problems; ↑ perinatal morbidity and mortality
- Older mothers: Down syndrome
- Obesity: ↑ gestational diabetes, ↑ perinatal mortality, ↑ difficult delivery
- Drug abuse: effects of drugs on foetus and newborn
- Viral infection; human immunodeficiency virus (HIV); hepatitis B and C.

Ideally, women should be in good health and prepared for pregnancy at the time of conception. The foetus may suffer long-term effects from early adverse influences (Figure 7.1).

7.3   Congenital malformations

About 2% of all babies are born with serious congenital defects, sufficient to threaten life, to cause permanent handicap or to require surgical correction (Table 7.1).

Distressingly, little is known of the causes of congenital abnormalities. Single-gene defects and chromosome anomalies account for 10–20% of the total. A small number are attributable to intrauterine infections (e.g. cytomegalovirus, rubella), fewer to teratogenic drugs and even fewer to ionizing radiation. The ideal is prevention.

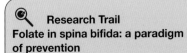
Research Trail
Folate in spina bifida: a paradigm of prevention

Laboratory and epidemiological studies showed the importance of folate. Increased folate intake reduces the incidence and prevents recurrence.

Next Research Trail on page 80

Nature protects against birth of children with serious anomalies. The incidence of serious defects and

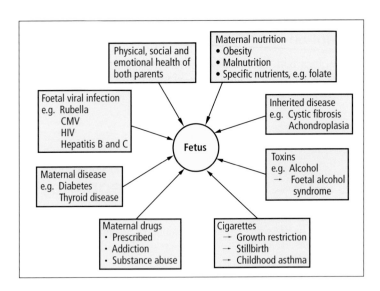

Figure 7.1 Factors affecting foetal nutrition, growth and development.

Table 7.1 Incidence of some congenital problems

Down syndrome	1 : 600
Club foot	1 : 700
Polydactyly/syndactyly	1 : 700
Cleft lip/palate	1 : 800
Congenital heart disease	1 : 1000
Spina bifida/anencephaly	1 : 2000
Oesophageal atresia	1 : 3000
Diaphragmatic hernia	1 : 3500

abortions is very high. It can be shown, for example, that at least 90% of embryos/foetuses with trisomy 21, and a much higher proportion of embryos with sex chromosome anomalies, are aborted. Live-born, malformed infants therefore represent the small minority of abnormal conceptuses.

PRACTICE POINT

It is important that pregnant women are advised to avoid all alcohol through the pregnancy due to the risk of foetal alcohol syndrome.

7.3.1 Prenatal diagnosis (Table 7.2)

Choice of technique for prenatal diagnosis is difficult. More invasive tests may provide more definitive information, but may risk precipitation of miscarriage. Amniocentesis has a 1% risk of miscarriage. Some foetal intervention is highly successful (e.g. foetal blood sampling or transfusion for anaemia or thrombocytopenia), while foetal surgery (e.g. relief of urinary obstruction or diaphragmatic hernia) remains experimental.

Reasons for prenatal diagnosis

- Reassurance of parents
- Management of pregnancy and delivery
- Selective termination of pregnancy
- Planned neonatal management
- Intrauterine treatment.

PRACTICE POINT
Screening for Down syndrome

- Ultrasound (increased nuchal thickness – the depth of the skin fold over the back of the neck)
- Quadruple test (maternal blood: ↓ α-fetoprotein, ↑ gonadotropin, ↓ oestriol and ↑ inhibin A)
- Karyotyping for trisomy 21 (chorionic villus sampling/amniocentesis).

Table 7.2 Modes of prenatal diagnosis

Mode	Type of investigation	Example
Ultrasound	Foetal measurement Foetal anomaly • Missing structures • Enlarged organs • Abnormalities	IUGR Anencephaly, renal agenesis Polycystic kidneys Cardiac Oligohydramnios: IUGR Polyhydramnios: oesophageal atresia
Amniocentesis	Fluid analysis Foetal cells	↑ Alpha-fetoprotein in spina bifida ↑ Bilirubin in haemolysis Karyotyping/DNA analysis
Maternal blood	Biochemistry	Quadruple test for Down syndrome
Chorionic villus sampling	Genetic testing/Karyotyping/DNA analysis	Down syndrome or cystic fibrosis
Fetoscopy, cordocentesis (foetal blood sampling)	Foetal blood and tissue	Wide variety of investigations

7.4 Embryonic and foetal growth and development

In early pregnancy, the embryological timetable determines teratogenic hazards. Infective, chemical or physical agents that cause birth defects may only be teratogenic at certain times in pregnancy. Rubella, for example, has devastating effects in the first trimester and almost none in the third trimester.

In the second and third trimesters, foetal growth, estimated clinically or by ultrasound, is an important indicator of foetal health. Ultrasound can also be used for fuller assessment of well-being (foetal biophysical profile). The healthy foetus shows normal growth, foetal breathing movements and good volume of amniotic fluid and has normal blood flow velocities measured in the foetal arteries by Doppler. Loss of these features implies foetal compromise and is useful in timing delivery.

The increase in size from conception to birth is phenomenal. At 8 weeks, all major organs have been formed. All serious congenital malformations have their origins in these early weeks. More serious malformations often result in early foetal death and spontaneous abortion.

At 8 weeks, the embryo, who only weighs 1 g, becomes a foetus. Weight gain accelerates, and at 24 weeks (the lower limit of viability), the foetus weighs just around 600 g. Weight gain increases through the final trimester to 100–250 g/week.

 Summary

Multidisciplinary care, supported by innovations in technology, has led to dramatic changes in our knowledge of foetal well-being and detection of abnormality. A healthy child with healthy, loving parents is the best outcome in every pregnancy. In your attachment to paediatrics or obstetrics, ask to attend foetal ultrasound and consider going to a foetal medicine clinic.

 FOR YOUR LOG

(Note that some items in this section may be more easily carried out in a clinical placement in Obstetrics and Gynaecology.)

- Understand the principle of Gillick competency and observe/reflect on scenarios where this applies.
- Observe a consultation where prenatal screening is discussed.
- Observe antenatal ultrasound.

See EMQ 7.1 at the end of the book.

SBAs

Q7.1 A raised alpha-fetoprotein level is detected in a maternal blood sample during pregnancy.
What can this be associated with?
a. Down syndrome
b. Edwards syndrome
c. Klinefelter syndrome
d. Patau syndrome
e. Spina bifida

Q7.2 On a newborn examination of a term baby, it is small for gestational age with microcephaly. You notice some facial features of a smooth philtrum, thin upper lip and mid-face hypoplasia. The red reflex is visible bilaterally, and there is no jaundice and no hepatosplenomegaly.
What is the most likely cause?
a. Congenital Rubella
b. Foetal alcohol syndrome
c. Folate deficiency
d. Gestational diabetes
e. Group B streptococcal infection

For SBA answers, see page 366.

The umbilical cord has two arteries and one vein. A single artery may be associated with congenital malformation. The cord is clamped about 1 cm from the skin surface and cut close to the clamp. The cord stump should be observed carefully for signs of infection. Staphylococcal infection is important but unusual.

Bathing. It is tempting to wash the newborn clean after birth, but bathing risks hypothermia and can be deferred for a few days. Vernix, a natural layer of grease which is present *in utero*, is absorbed naturally.

Passage of meconium and urine. It is important to note the time of first passing meconium and urine, and often, this occurs at or soon after delivery. Both are usually passed within 24 h of birth, and delay should prompt a search for underlying pathology.

Feeding. This topic is dealt with fully in Sections 13.1 and 13.3. The ideal is to put the baby to the breast shortly after birth. The first feed, of either breast milk or a formula, should be offered within 6 h of birth.

8.4 Examination of the newborn

All newborn babies should have a clinical examination in the first 24 h. The mother should be present, and in the vast majority, it will be possible to reassure parents that all is well.

PRACTICE POINT

The aims of newborn examinations are to:
- Detect conditions that:
  - Will benefit from early treatment
  - Need long-term supervision
  - Have genetic implications
  - Indicate systemic illness.
- Discuss parental anxieties and take a brief medical, genetic and social history, seeking information that may be relevant to the future health and development of the baby.
- Provide advice on matters such as infant feeding, attendance at baby clinics and immunization.
- Advise on minor abnormalities which may lead to worry.

8.4.1 Suggested scheme for routine clinical examination

General observation. Does the infant look well? Is she pink and responsive? Is she tachypnoeic or pale?

Check for the normal flexed posture and symmetrical limb movements. Are there dysmorphic features? Look for cyanosis, jaundice, skin rashes and birthmarks.

Measurements. Check weight and occipitofrontal head circumference for gestational age on a centile chart.

Head. Check head shape. Moulding (change of head shape during delivery) is common and resolves in days. Assess the tension of the anterior fontanelle and the width of the sutures. These vary greatly between babies, but a full fontanelle with wide sutures may indicate hydrocephalus.

Face. Has the baby got a normal face or any dysmorphic features? Is there a facial nerve palsy?

Eyes. Simply look carefully at the eyes and make sure there is a red reflex (excluding cataract or retinoblastoma) (Section 3.5.6.8, p. 44). Asymmetry of eye size is abnormal: small eyes may occur in congenital viral infection or developmental defect, or one eye may be

---

Common conditions of little clinical importance

Skin lesions
- Strawberry naevi (Figure 25.3)
- 'Stork' marks (Figure 25.1)
- Milia (small collections in the sebaceous glands which disappear soon after birth) (Figure 8.4)
- Erythema toxicum (a blotchy red rash; each spot has a yellow centre which is full of eosinophils. Spots come and go. It is benign and should be distinguished from skin sepsis)
- Slate grey naevi (mongolian blue spots) (Section 25.1.2.2)
- Epithelial 'pearls' (small white cysts near the midline on the palate)

Subconjunctival haemorrhage

Cephalohaematoma (Figure 8.5) – see 'Soft tissue injuries' later in this chapter

Positional talipes (you need to distinguish from structural talipes that needs surgery (Section 24.1.6)

Peripheral and traumatic cyanosis (blue hands and feet are normal in the first days. Facial congestion looks like cyanosis)

Breast enlargement (due to maternal oestrogen; this resolves with time)

Oral and vulval mucosal tags

Sacral dimple (extremely rarely connects with spinal cord but make sure you can see the bottom of the dimple)

Skin tags and diminutive accessory digits.

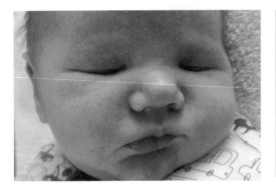

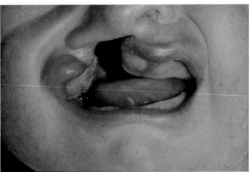

Figure 8.4 Milia. Small raised, white spots over the nose and cheeks. This baby also has two erythema toxicum spots on the right eyelid.

Figure 8.6 Unilateral cleft lip and palate.

cavity should be checked for the presence of teeth, cysts or thrush (candida infection).

Jaw. A small or recessed mandible (retrognathia) can lead to feeding difficulty or respiratory obstruction.

Chest. Check the baby is pink and not breathless.

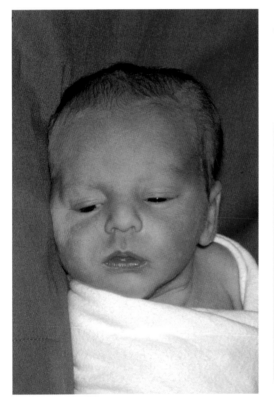

Figure 8.5 Unilateral cephalohaematoma.

large (congenital glaucoma). The eye should be checked for signs of infection.

Mouth. The palate should be inspected for clefts and palpated for submucosal clefts (Figure 8.6). The oral

---

Primitive reflexes

Grasp – birth to 4 months The infant grasps an object placed in palm or under toes.

Moro (startle) reflex – birth to 4 months
- Hold the infant supporting the head and allow the head to drop gently a few centimetres. The infant will look surprised or even cry, throw its arms outwards and then bring them back to the midline. Explain what you are doing to the mother.

Asymmetric tonic neck reflex (ATNR) – birth to 7 months
- On turning the head to one side, the ipsilateral arm and leg are extended.

Rooting reflex – from birth
- On touching the infant's face, he turns, opening his mouth as if to suck on the finger.

Persistence of the Moro and ATNR is abnormal and may indicate cerebral palsy.

Heart. Which side is the heart best heard on? Where is the apex beat? Heart murmurs are very common in babies and most relate to the transition from foetal to adult circulatory pattern and disappear in the first days. It is difficult to tell which murmurs are significant, and it is important not to worry parents unnecessarily. Pansystolic, diastolic or very loud murmurs are likely to be important.

Abdomen. The liver edge is usually palpable 1–2 cm below the right costal margin, and the spleen can be tipped in at least 20% of normal babies. The lower poles of both kidneys may be palpable.

Groin. Absent femoral pulses may denote coarctation of the aorta. Check for hernias.

Genitalia. Check that the genitalia are clearly either male or female. If there is doubt, do not ascribe sex. In boys, check that the testes are in the scrotum and that the urethral meatus is where it should be. In girls, inspect the genitalia and remember that a little vaginal bleeding or discharge of clear mucus is normal secondary to the influence of maternal and placental hormones.

Anus. Ask if the baby has passed meconium, and check that the anus is present, patent and normally located.

Spine. Turn the baby prone. Inspect the entire spine for lumps, naevi, hairy patches, pits or sinuses which may indicate spinal cord abnormality.

Hips. Examination of the hips is very important (Section 24.1.7). It is best left to the end of the examination as it may upset the baby.

Central nervous system. Is the baby moving spontaneously? Is there symmetry of movement? Are limbs held in the usual flexed position? Ask about feeding behaviour. Assess tone by picking the baby up and holding her in ventral suspension. Elicit the Moro reflex (see above, this chapter, 'Primitive reflexes').

Biochemical screening. Routine screening on blood spot tests (the Guthrie card) is carried out on days 5–7 for hypothyroidism (Section 28.3), cystic fibrosis (Section 20.8), haemoglobinopathy (Section 26.2.2.1) and inherited metabolic conditions such as phenylketonuria (Section 28.7.1) and medium-chain acyl-CoA dehydrogenase deficiency (MCADD) (Section 28.7.2).

8.5   Birth injury (physical trauma)

Serious birth injury is rare. Tentorial tears (injury to the fold of dura between the cerebrum and cerebellum) can be fatal or lead to permanent cerebral damage, but are hardly ever seen now. Minor trauma is quite commonly discovered on routine examination. Trauma is more common after obstructed labour (due to a small pelvis or a large baby), precipitate labour, malpresentation and heroic instrumental delivery.

8.5.1   Nerve palsies

Most lesions recover as traumatic swelling subsides, but minor disability persists in about 15%, and a few are left handicapped.

8.5.1.1   Brachial plexus palsies

These usually follow the difficult delivery of a big

 PRACTICE POINT

Erb's palsy (Figure 8.7) affects C5/6 roots, resulting in weakness or paralysis. The affected arm lies straight and limp beside the trunk. The forearm is internally rotated and with the fingers flexed (waiter's tip position). When the Moro reflex is elicited, the affected arm does not respond.

baby.
   Rarely, the lower roots C8/T1 are injured, resulting in weakness of wrist extensors and intrinsic muscles of the hand (*Klumpke's palsy*).

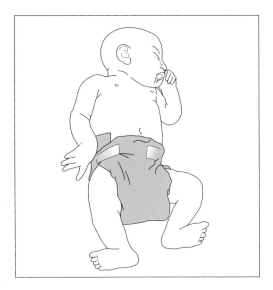

Figure 8.7 Erb's palsy.

8.5.1.2   Facial nerve palsy

The facial nerve may be injured by pressure from the maternal pelvic bones or by forceps blades. It is a lower motor neurone defect, usually unilateral.

8.5.1.3   Phrenic nerve palsy

Rarely, the cervical roots of the phrenic nerve are damaged, causing diaphragmatic paralysis and respiratory difficulty.

8.5.2   Skeletal injury

8.5.2.1   Clavicle fracture

This commonly follows shoulder dystocia. Complete breaks are painful and limit the baby's arm movements. Clavicle fractures heal well, but often with considerable callus formation.

8.5.2.2   Humerus and femur

Fractures and epiphyseal injury may rarely occur during difficult births. They heal well.

8.5.2.3   Skull fractures

The compliant skull of the newborn is remarkably resistant to fracture. Asymptomatic linear fractures of the parietal bone are most common. Depressed fractures require surgical elevation.

8.5.3   Soft tissue injuries

8.5.3.1   Cephalohaematoma

PRACTICE POINT

In a cephalohaematoma, the swelling and amount of blood loss are limited by the periosteum attached to the margins of the skull bone so it does not cross the midline (Figure 8.5).

A cephalohaematoma caused by subperiosteal bleeding is common, occurring in 1–2%. It may make jaundice worse as the blood in it is reabsorbed. Infection may occur if the skin is broken. The vast majority resolve spontaneously, although the edge may calcify.

8.5.3.2   Subaponeurotic haemorrhage

Haemorrhage between the periosteum and galea aponeurotica (a thick membrane going from the eyebrows to the occiput) is potentially lethal. The space is not limited like a cephalohaematoma, and serious blood loss can occur. It is more common after ventouse delivery. The baby appears pale with a raised fluctuant swelling of the scalp.

8.5.3.3   Sternomastoid tumour

This is a fusiform fibrous mass in the middle of the sternomastoid muscle. It may follow trauma. It usually disappears over about 6 months. Gentle physiotherapy to prevent shortening of the muscle is required.

8.5.3.4   Bruising and abrasions

Difficult births are often accompanied by bruising. Usually, there is little serious harm. Breakdown of extravasated blood may contribute to neonatal jaundice. Skin abrasions are portals of entry for microorganisms and should be observed for signs of infection.

8.6   Congenital malformations

Congenital abnormalities are an important cause of perinatal mortality and short- and long-term morbidity (Figure 8.8). Most of the common defects are

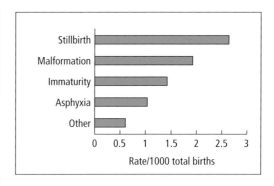

Figure 8.8 Causes of perinatal death (the stillbirth rate is for foetuses without abnormality).

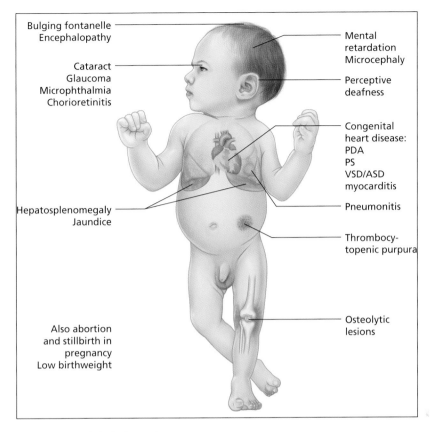

Bulging fontanelle
Encephalopathy

Mental
retardation
Microcephaly

Cataract
Glaucoma
Microphthalmia
Chorioretinitis

Perceptive
deafness

Congenital
heart disease:
PDA
PS
VSD/ASD
myocarditis

Pneumonitis

Hepatosplenomegaly
Jaundice

Thrombocy-
topenic purpura

Osteolytic
lesions

Also abortion
and stillbirth in
pregnancy
Low birthweight

Figure 9.9 Features of congenital rubella syndrome.

- Pneumonia and/or meningitis due to GBS
- *E. coli* septicaemia and/or meningitis
- Gonococcal and chlamydia eye infection
- Herpes simplex.

9.4.4.3 Infection acquired after birth

Once born, the baby rapidly becomes colonized by bacteria and usually this occurs without harm. Infection is especially likely if colonization is heavy or if the organisms are of high pathogenicity. Organisms in the blood stream may give rise to septicaemia, meningitis or pneumonia.

Any baby with suspected infection should be examined carefully. Perform an infection screen: full blood count, blood culture, chest X-ray, microscopy and culture of urine and cerebrospinal fluid (CSF). Immediate investigation and antibiotic may be life-saving. GBS (see above) is the commonest and most important infection, while other common organisms are *E. coli, Staphylococcus aureus* and *Listeria*. Coagulase-negative staphylococcus is the most common pathogen in the preterm infant.

 PRACTICE POINT   **Common early signs of infection**

- Lethargy and hypotonia
- Poor feeding, abdominal distension or vomiting
- Pallor and mottling of the skin
- Disturbed temperature regulation
- Tachypnoea or recurrent apnoea.

 TREATMENT

Do not wait for results – if infection is suspected give broad-spectrum antibiotics, typically benzylpenicillin and gentamicin.

9.4.4.4 Sticky eye

The cause of most sticky eyes is poor drainage down the nasolacrimal duct. Often all that is necessary is to bathe the eye with warm saline. More serious eye infections may be due to staphylococci and coliforms.

9.4.4.5   Skin infection

Septic spots and paronychia, usually due to staphylococcal infection, are relatively common and responsive to local treatment, but may need systemic antibiotics.

PRACTICE POINT

If a baby has severe purulent eye infection in the first 10 days, this is typical of gonococcus or *Chlamydia trachomatis* infection. Urgent diagnosis and treatment are needed.

9.4.4.6   Candida infection

Infection of the mouth and nappy area by yeasts is common. It responds well to nystatin or miconazole. Therapy should be continued for a few days longer than it takes to clear the signs of infection. Hygiene of bottles and dummies must be scrupulous.

9.4.5   Convulsions

Convulsions occurring in the first days of life have many causes. Perinatal brain injury is important. Severe seizures are a poor prognostic sign.

Seizures always require immediate and thorough investigation and treatment of any underlying disorder. If the cause cannot be remedied, anticonvulsant medication is given.

Causes of seizures

- Intrapartum asphyxia
- Intracranial bleeds
- Hypoglycaemia
- Meningitis
- Low Ca or Mg
- Inborn error of metabolism
- Brain malformation or abnormality

 # Summary

Most problems in the preterm infant are due to organ immaturity and are closely linked to gestation. Each week below 32 weeks increases the chance of serious problems. The outlook for the preterm infant has improved massively in the last few decades. In the infant who is SGA, problems relate to the cause of the LBW and to poor foetal nutrition. In the term infant who becomes unwell, always consider infection and hypoglycaemia, especially in high-risk infants. Every baby that is successfully treated acquires over 70 quality-adjusted life years.

FOR YOUR LOG

- Visit the neonatal intensive care ward. Ask to join the ward round. Go there when you are on call.
- Look at the chest X-ray of a baby with RDS.
- Make sure you have seen an apnoea monitor and know how to set it.
- See a baby having phototherapy.

See EMQ 9.1, EMQ 9.2, EMQ 9.3 and EMQ 9.4 at the end of the book.

SBAs

Q9.1 A newborn breastfed baby girl that is 12 hours old is noted to be jaundiced. What is the most likely cause?
a.   Breast milk jaundice
b.   Extrahepatic biliary atresia
c.   Physiological jaundice
d.   Rhesus haemolytic disease
e.   Sickle cell disease

Q9.2 A 2-day-old baby is noted to be pyrexial and irritable. There is a history of maternal pyrexia in labour and prolonged rupture of membranes lasting 26 h. What is the most appropriate treatment?
a.   Benzylpenicillin and Gentamicin
b.   Ceftriaxone
c.   Cefuroxime
d.   Flucloxacillin
e.   Observation on neonatal unit

For SBA answers, see page 366.

Child development and how to assess it

Chapter map

Child development is the gradual acquisition of new skills and behaviours through childhood. Knowledge of development helps you to understand the presentation and impact of illness in children and will help you to adapt your history and examination for age. In this chapter, we describe normal development and a practical approach to assessment.

Healthy development has a wide range of 'normal'.

10.1 Normal development

Development is normally divided into several separate areas; learn these for a systematic approach, but be flexible.

> **PRACTICE POINT** **Development is categorized into four areas**
>
> - Gross motor – Posture and movement
> - Fine motor and vision
> - Speech and language – Including hearing
> - Social – behaviour and play

10.1.1 Range of normal

The age at which a normal child achieves a particular physical or developmental goal is extremely variable; 50% of children can walk 10 steps unaided at 13 months, but a few can do this at 8 months and others not until 18 months. It is best to talk to parents of the 'usual' age for developing a skill rather than the 'normal', since abnormal implies problems. Quite commonly one field of activity appears delayed in a normal child, but it is rare for all four fields of development to be delayed if the child is normal. In the preterm infant, the correct age for gestation before assessing development.

Delayed development that is following a normal sequence is likely to be normal unless the delay is severe. Bizarre and unusual patterns of development are more worrying.

Paediatrics Lecture Notes, Tenth Edition. Jonathan C. Darling and James Yong.
© 2022 John Wiley & Sons Ltd. Published 2022 by John Wiley & Sons Ltd.
Companion website: www.wiley.com/go/lecturenotes/paediatrics10e

10.1.2 Milestones are stepping stones

Parents tend to think of certain developmental skills as essential milestones. It is truer to regard them as stepping stones. In general, one cannot reach a particular stepping stone without using the previous ones – and a child does not run until she can walk, or walk until she can stand. However, different people may use different stepping stones, and occasionally miss one out. Most children crawl before they stand, but some shuffle on their bottoms, never crawl, yet stand and walk normally in the end. *Bottom shuffling* is a typical example of the sort of variation in development that can cause parents unnecessary worry, particularly as bottom shufflers tend to walk later than other children.

Using stepping stones, we may go in sudden bounds rather than at an even rate – children often develop that way, appearing static for a few weeks then suddenly mastering a new skill. If the next stepping stone is a particularly hard one, all the child's energy may appear to be devoted to just one of the four areas of development, whilst the other three seem static; posture and movement skills may advance rapidly about the age of 1 year as walking is mastered, whilst hearing and speech development appear static.

Whether we like it or not, many parents view their child's developmental assessment in the same way as an undergraduate examination, and all parents want their child to 'pass'. Therefore:

- When we 'test' beyond expected skills – reassure that we do not expect the 9- to 12-month-old child to walk.
- Announce 'results' early – if development is normal, say so.
- Handle 'failure' carefully – be sure before you diagnose developmental delay.

10.2 Developmental assessment

There are two purposes of developmental assessment:

- Early detection of significant delay so that help (advice, physiotherapy, spectacles, hearing aid) can be provided early.
- To provide reassurance to parents.

There are two parts to developmental assessment:

- History
- Observation

The history is usually reliable and augments the clinical examination. Parents may exaggerate their child's abilities or misinterpret involuntary movements.

10.2.1 History

- Ask in detail about presentation skills.
- Cover the four main categories.
- How do these compare with those of older siblings at that age? (This may influence parents' perceptions.)
- School performance (if at school) – a significant developmental problem is unlikely if the child is coping well in a normal class.
- Past history – especially dates of early milestones.
- Some parents recall milestones well, others not at all. Many have documented them in the parent-held record. If an experienced parent says 'she was very quick', it may not be necessary to obtain exact detail of past achievements.

10.2.2 Observation

- Play with the child in the presence of the parent.
- Demonstrate each skill where possible.
- Define the limit of achievement by noting both the skills the child has and those he has not.

You can easily carry out the following simple tests in any surgery or clinic. No special equipment or expertise is needed. They are screening tests which identify children who need more detailed expert assessment. The ages given are the average ages at which the skill is seen.

 PRACTICE POINT **The first 6 months**

This is the most difficult time to assess the baby, because it is not until about 6 months that many of the easier developmental tests can be used. Therefore, developmental testing before the age of 6 months is less reliable than at any other time.

10.2.3 Gross motor – Posture and movement

Body control is acquired from the top downwards:

- Head on trunk – the newborn baby held upright can balance his head briefly but laid on his back and pulled up by arms or shoulders, there is complete head lag. By 4 months, the head comes up in line with the trunk. By 6 months, the head comes up in advance of the trunk.
- Trunk on pelvis – by 6 months a baby can sit supported on a firm, flat surface, but left will topple over (do not let this happen). By 8–9 months, he sits without arm support and can turn without falling.
- Pelvis on legs – by 9 months he will weight bear and helps to stand up. At 10 months, he is pulling himself up to stand and cruising (walking holding on) round the furniture. By 12 months, he can take some steps unaided.

10.2.4 Fine motor and vision

10.2.4.1 Visual attention

- At 8 weeks, a baby observes with a convergent gaze a dangling toy or bright object held 20–30 cm (9–12 inches) from his face and moves his head and neck in order to follow it.
- From 2 months, a baby prefers to watch a face rather than anything else. The ability to fix and follow improves and can be tested by watching the baby follow a rolling ball, the toddler matching toys (Figure 10.1) or the 5-year-old matching letters.

> **PRACTICE POINT**
>
> Babies may squint transiently in the first 3 months, but a persisting true squint (as distinct from a pseudo-squint as seen with epicanthic folds) is always abnormal and requires referral to a specialist (see Chapter 11).

10.2.4.2 Grasp and pincer grip

Palmar grasp

- Offer a large object
  - A wooden tongue depressor
  - A 2.5 cm cube

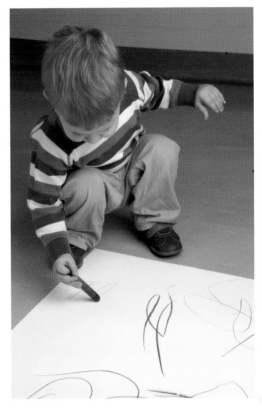

Figure 10.1 Ask the child to draw and copy shapes with a crayon.

- Observe how it is grasped
  - At 6 months, there is a clumsy palmar grasp, object approached with the ulnar border of the hand.
  - At 9 months, he approaches it with the radial border and takes it in a scissor grasp between the sides of thumb and index finger before transferring it to the other hand and putting in his mouth.
  - At 12 months, he approaches it with the index finger and picks it up precisely between the ends of the thumb and index finger in a pincer grasp.

Pincer grip

- Offer a small object, e.g. a sultana (check with parents first). Observe for an index finger approach (9 months) and a pincer grasp (9–12 months).
- Once this is developed, parents notice that their child can pick up the tiniest bits of fluff on the carpet (Figure 10.2).

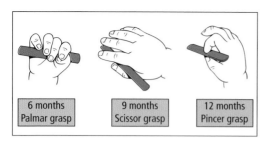

| 6 months | 9 months | 12 months |
| Palmar grasp | Scissor grasp | Pincer grasp |

Figure 10.2 Development of grasp.

 PRACTICE POINT

Do not expose the child to danger during developmental assessment. Children may choke on small objects. Scissors are perilous.

10.2.5 Speech and language

10.2.5.1 Localization of sounds (distraction test)

The baby is sat on the parent's knee facing another adult about 3 m (10 feet) away whose function is to keep the baby's visual attention straight ahead (but without being so fascinating that the baby ignores the test sounds).

A variety of quiet, soft sounds are made lateral to either ear and out of the line of vision. Rustling tissue provides a high-frequency sound; a spoon gently scraped round a cup, or a high-pitched rattle is other suitable sounds. Provided the baby has reasonable hearing, she will turn to locate the source. At 7 months, the baby turns to sounds 0.5 m from either ear. At 9 months, he turns promptly to sounds 1 m away. The optimal age at which to test an infant's hearing is 7 months.

The distraction test used to be a child's first screening hearing test, but there have been concerns about how well it performs. Neonatal screening of hearing is now used in the UK, and routine distraction testing is not necessary.

10.2.5.2 Speech

3 months – open vowel sounds (ooh, eeh) – cooing
6 months – consonants (goo, gah) – gurgling
9 months – varied and tuneful babbling
1 year – single word labels used for familiar objects and people – 'Mum', 'Dog'
2 years – words joined to convey ideas – 'Dadad gone' – child follows simple instructions, e.g. 'Put the spoon in the cup'
3 years – sentences used to describe present and past happenings.

Throughout this period, the child's understanding of language is far ahead of his ability to utter it.

10.2.6 Social behaviour

10.2.6.1 Smiling

Seen at 4–8 weeks in response to mother's face.

10.2.6.2 Reacting to strangers

Up to 9 months, most babies will be handled happily by anyone; from 9 months, they begin to cry or fret if handled by a stranger.

10.2.6.3 Feeding

At 9 months, lumpy food is chewed. At 18 months, the child cooperates with feeding, and drinks from an ordinary cup using two hands. At 3 years, he can feed himself efficiently with a spoon and fork (Table 10.1).

 PRACTICE POINT

Table 10.1 shows median ages for developmental milestones which are useful to remember. However, there are upper age ranges by which a child should have achieved certain developmental milestones or it may indicate a 'red flag' and require further investigation.

An example of this is the median age for starting to walk alone may be 12 months. If a child is not walking by 18 months, they will need to be assessed and investigated.

Table 10.1 Developmental milestones (average age of achievements)

Age	Gross motor	Fine motor and vision	Hearing and speech	Social
6–8 weeks	Briefly hold head up when held prone	Vision: fixes and follows through 90°	Vocalizes	Smiles responsively
3–4 months	Prone: rests on forearms, lifts up head and chest Pulled to sit: head bobs forwards, then held erect Rolls over	Vision: fixes and follows through 180° Hands: loosely open	Chuckles and coos when pleased Quietens to interesting sounds	Laughs Regards own hands
6 months	Sits – erect with support (unsupported 8–9 months) Prone: lifts up on extended arms Held standing: takes weight on legs	Reaches out for toy and takes in palmar grasp, puts to mouth Transfers object from hand to hand Watches rolling ball 2 m away	Makes double syllable sounds and tuneful noises (gurgles) Localizes soft sounds 45 cm (15 inches) lateral to either ear	Alert, interested Still friendly with strangers
9–10 months	Crawls Walks around furniture stepping sideways (cruising)	Scissor grasp Looks for toys that are dropped	Babbles tunefully Brisk localisation of soft sounds 1 m lateral to either ear	Distinguishes strangers and shows apprehension Chews solids
12 months	Walks a few steps alone	Index finger approach to tiny objects then pincer grasp Drops toys deliberately and watches where they go	Babbles incessantly A few words Understands simple commands	Cooperates with dressing, e.g. holding up arms Waves bye bye
18 months	Walks well and can pick up a toy from floor without falling	Builds tower of three cubes Scribbles	Uses many words, sound labels Occasionally two words together	Drinks from cup using two hands Demands constant mothering
2 years	Runs Walks up and down stairs two feet to a step	Builds tower of six cubes	Joins words together in simple phrases, as sound ideas	Uses spoon Indicates toilet needs, dry by day Play imitates adult activities
3 years	Walks upstairs one foot per step, and down two feet per step Rides tricycle	Builds tower of nine cubes Copies O	Speaks in sentences Gives full name	Eats with spoon and fork Can undress with assistance Dry by night
4 years	Walks up and down stairs one foot per step Stands on one foot for 5 s	Builds three steps from six cubes (after demonstration) Copies O and +	Talks a lot Speech contains many infantile substitutions	Dresses and undresses with assistance
5 years	Skips, hops Stands on one foot with arms folded for 5 s	Draws a man Copies O, + and □	Fluent speech with few infantile substitutions	Dresses and undresses alone Washes and dries face and hands

10.3   Notes and memory aids

 PRACTICE POINT   **Notes and memory aids** (Figure 10.3)

Small wooden 2.5 cm (1 inch) cubes are best.

The tower of bricks is roughly three times the age in years (between 1.5 and 3 years) (Figure 10.4).

A cross is part of the figure '4' and is copied at 4 years.

Age 3 is the age of '3's and circles:

- The bridge at age 3 has 3 bricks, the tower 3 × 3 bricks.
- A 3-year-old kicks a ball, draws a circle, rides a trike (three wheels), knows (at least) three body parts and three colours and speaks in (at least) three-word sentences.

Age (yr)	Tower of bricks (number of bricks in a tower)	Shape with bricks	Copying shapes
1.5	3		
2	6		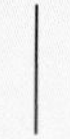 |
2.5		Train 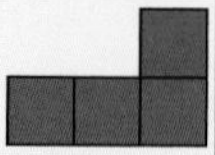	
3	9	Bridge 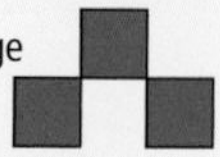	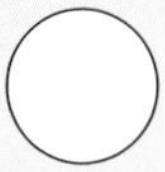 ◯
4	-	Steps 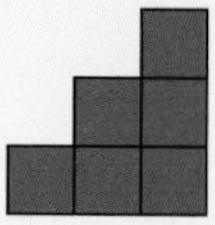	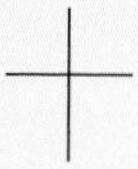 +
5	-		▢

Figure 10.3 Assessing fine motor development. Small wooden 2.5 cm (1 inch) cubes are best for tower building and brick shapes. Ask the child to copy the shapes.

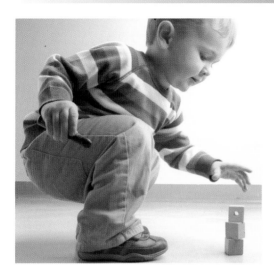

Figure 10.4 Small bricks (for tower-building and shapes) are used to assess fine motor skills.

10.4 Limitations of developmental assessment

The range of normal means assessment cannot be too precise. Aim to give a range of a few months for each area. Practice improves the reliability of assessment, but simply listening to the parents and observing the child will provide useful information in the four main fields of development. If the parents' account differs greatly from what is observed, it may be that the child is having an 'off day', in which case observing on another occasion will be more reliable.

 PRACTICE POINT

Remember that all 'candidates' can have an off day – interpretation is difficult during illness.

 Summary

Developmental assessment is a key skill in paediatrics. Use the 'four areas' to help you, and build-up an understanding of normal sequences that run through each.

 FOR YOUR LOG

- Do developmental assessments on children aged about 6 months, 12 months and 18 months.
- Observe normal child development and behaviour in a preschool or nursery setting.

 OSCE TIP

- A child of up to 2 years with normal development (see OSCE Station 10.1).
- A video of a child with developmental delay.
- A child with Down syndrome with global developmental delay.
- A child who is deaf with speech and language delay.

See EMQ 10.1 and EMQ 10.2 at the end of the book.

OSCE station 10.1: Developmental assessment

Clinical approach:

- Combine history, observation and clinical testing
  - ◇ Watch the child playing
  - ◇ Think of four areas of development
- Assessment of four areas:
  - ◇ **Gross motor**
  - ◇ **Fine motor and vision**
  - ◇ **Hearing and speech**
  - ◇ **Social**
- Think in 3-month intervals
- In each area of development:
  - ◇ Find a skill that the child can do
  - ◇ Find a more advanced skill that the child cannot do
  - ◇ Developmental age is between the two
- Use any set of recognized milestones
- Present findings for each area of development
- Summarize your findings

This is Rachel and her mother. Please perform a developmental assessment and tell me how old she is

Posture and movement

sits supported rolls over
NOT cruising
NOT walking

Vision and manipulation

index approach scissor grip transfers
NOT pincer grip

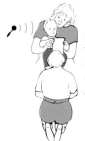

Hearing and Speech

passed health visitor test turns to sound babbles – lots of sounds
NO words

Social/personal

waves bye holds, bites, chews biscuit holds bottle when feeding
NOT handing things back
STILL mouthing
Rachel is a healthy child of 10 months

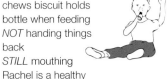

Never forget:

- Say hello and introduce yourself
- General health – is the child ill?
- Quickly assess growth, nutrition and development
- Mention the obvious (e.g. bandage on arm)

Look around for:

- Walking aids
- Hearing aids, evidence of feeding problems
- Glasses
- Adapted buggy

Special points

- Praise the things a child can do and reassure them when they cannot perform
- Developmental age may not be the same in each of the four areas – this can be normal
- Did the child perform to her ability?
- Children in the developmental OSCE are usually normal healthy children
- As soon as development is considered, start observing the child – they may perform brilliantly until you begin a formal assessment, and then go on strike!

SBAs

Q10.1   A 20-month-old boy is not yet walking. On examination, he is not able to get up from a supine position without rolling onto his front and using his hands to 'climb up' his legs. He has hypertrophy of his calf muscles.
What is the most useful initial investigation?

a.   Creatinine kinase
b.   Karyotype
c.   MRI head
d.   MRI spine
e.   Muscle biopsy

Q10.2   A 4-week-old baby has multiple rib fractures, retinal haemorrhages and subdural haemorrhages. They have presented with a history of rolling off the bed onto a carpeted floor.
What is the most likely cause?

a.   Haemophilia A
b.   Idiopathic Thrombocytopenia Purpura
c.   Non-accidental injury
d.   Osteogenesis imperfecta
e.   Vitamin D deficiency rickets

For SBA answers, see page 366.

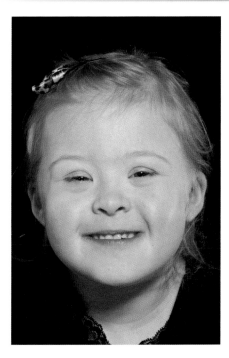

Figure 11.2 A child with Down syndrome.

carried by a parent giving a high risk of recurrence (Section 6.2.1).

Prenatal diagnosis (Section 7.3.1) has made little impression on the birth prevalence of the condition, since it is partly counterbalanced by increasing maternal age. The news of an unexpected diagnosis on the day of birth can be devastating for a family and demand senior and skilled handling (Section 2.2.3.1).

Although none of the characteristic features of Down syndrome is pathognomonic, and any may be present in a normal child, the association of several features usually enables a clinical diagnosis to be made (Figure 11.2). Recognition in very small preterm babies is difficult, and the condition is easily overlooked in aborted foetuses.

11.3.1.1   Diagnosis

This can usually be made with confidence on clinical grounds but should be confirmed by chromosome analysis (karyotype, Figure 11.1), which is also necessary for genetic counselling.

11.3.1.2   Progress

Apart from any problems arising from associated congenital abnormalities, babies with Down syndrome may be difficult to feed in the early weeks. Thereafter,

Features

- Eyes
  - *Oblique palpebral fissures*
  - *Prominent epicanthic folds*
  - *Brushfield spots* – tiny pale spots on the iris from infancy
- Head and face
  - *Brachycephalic skull* – face and occiput are flattened
  - *Third fontanelle* – at birth, between the anterior and posterior fontanelles
  - *Mouth* small and drooping
  - *Tongue* – becomes large and furrowed, often protrudes after infancy
  - *Pinna* may be abnormal in shape and low-set
  - *Neck* – short and broad, with excess skin posteriorly (the nuchal fold used in foetal screening)
- Hands and feet
  - *Hands and fingers* short and stubby
  - Single transverse palmar crease
  - *Clinodactyly* – short, incurved little finger
  - *Sandal gap* – wide gap between the first and second toes
- General
  - *Short stature* (there are Down centile charts)
  - *Hypotonicity* (floppiness) is always present
  - *Delayed development* in all aspects
  - Associated congenital abnormalities:
  - *Congenital heart disease* in 50% (usually atrioventricular septal defect)
  - *Duodenal atresia* and *congenital leukaemia* are associated, but much less common
- Long term
  - Increased risk of infections
  - Increased risk of leukaemia
  - Increased risk of thyroid problems and diabetes
  - Presenile dementia

they tend to be placid and to thrive, although they have an excess of respiratory tract infections. Most have moderately severe learning difficulties and require special educational help, but usually in their local school. As adults, they require continuing supervision. Their life expectancy is somewhat shorter than normal because of degenerative disorders of advancing age which develop a decade or two earlier than usual. Libido is diminished. Males have low fertility, females are fertile.

11.3.2   X-linked disability

Fragile X syndrome is the second most common genetic cause of severe learning disability; Down syndrome is the most common. More men than women are affected by a non-specific learning disability.

Fragile X syndrome

- Cognitive: moderate-to-severe learning difficulties
- Speech and language delay
- Behaviour: autistic features; aggression
- Physical: long thin face, big jaw, macroorchidism.

Fragile X syndrome is due to a triplet repeat on the X chromosome (Section 6.2.2.1, p. 68). The excess genetic material makes the area unstable when grown in special medium in the laboratory, hence the name.

Boys are most affected. Women may carry the condition or are affected less severely due to random inactivation of one of the X chromosomes. A positive family history is an important clue to the diagnosis.

11.3.3   Microcephaly

Primary microcephaly is associated with an inadequately developed brain at birth. The head circumference is small and falls further below the normal centiles. The fontanelles close early. In severe cases, the infant has a characteristic appearance: the face is normal but the skull vault is disproportionately small. Some cases are genetic (autosomal recessive). Others are caused by intrauterine infections (rubella, cytomegalovirus), toxins (alcohol) or (rarely) radiation. If the brain is damaged in the perinatal period, the poor head growth will become evident later.

Microcephaly must not be confused with craniosynostosis (Section 18.10.1). This is a disorder of fusion of sutures which will only result in a small head if it is neglected.

11.3.4   Disorders of speech and language

Normal language development varies considerably (Section 10.1). Children who are late in beginning to talk, or whose speech is thought to be abnormal, need careful assessment. Most will, in fact, go on to normal development. Some children have a sizeable vocabulary before their first birthday while others say little until 3 or 4 years old. A lisp is a common phase of speech development. Many 3- and 4-year-olds trip over their words because their thoughts and questions tumble out of their minds more quickly than they can articulate them. The average 4-year-old asks 26 questions an hour!

Significantly delayed or abnormal speech may be helped by early intervention. It is often helpful to refer any child with a speech problem to a speech therapist so that parents can be advised how best to help. The wrong kind of intervention may make the problem worse. There is a strong link between language delay and later educational difficulties.

If speech development is delayed:

- Is the child being spoken to? Speech is learned by imitation.
- Can the child hear? Deafness is an important cause of speech delay.
- Are other spheres of development delayed? If so, learning disability must be considered.
- Is there evidence of emotional/behavioural disorder? Late speech is usual in autism (Section 12.5.3.1) and fragile X.

The main abnormalities of speech are disorders of fluency (stammer/stutter) and of articulation. *Stammering* is common in young children and is much more common in boys than in girls. It usually goes spontaneously especially if it is ignored. If it persists into school age, it becomes a barrier to communication and a social embarrassment. Speech therapy is very effective.

Articulation disorders are common in young children. If they persist or are severe, the child may be

---

Speech problems

- Consonant substitution (e.g. 'Come' is pronounced 'Tum')
- Nasality, resulting from cleft palate or nasopharyngeal incompetence
- True dysarthria, as in some kinds of cerebral palsy (Section 18.8)
- Faulty enunciation, e.g. normal, orthodontic.

---

unintelligible. Speech therapy is essential for assessment and treatment. Occasionally, palatal or oral surgery is helpful.

11.4   School difficulties

If a healthy child of normal intelligence and good vision and hearing has educational difficulties, an emotional problem will often be found. There may be unhappiness at home, or at school (from bullying or fear), or family overexpectation or indifference.

Conversely, emotional problems may be the result of learning problems. A report from the school is an important part of the assessment of the schoolchild. More detailed assessment of intelligence and abilities by an educational psychologist will provide recommendations for remedial help.

Reasons for poor performance at school

Social/cultural
- Absence of family support for child and school
- Truancy
- Bullying, problems at school
- Poor home support for the child's study.

Neurological/psychological
- Major learning disability – usually detected before school
- Hearing, vision, fine motor, perceptive skills – often not detected.

Chronic ill health (any condition)
- Aim is to minimize effect on education.

School refusal (school phobia).

Learning problems: information needed

Clinical assessment
- Chronic illness
- Neurodevelopment
- Emotional problems
- Socioeconomic difficulties.

School report

Educational psychology

Vision and hearing.

11.4.1 Reading problems

Some children are much worse at reading, speech and language than at other skills, and remedial therapy is difficult. This is more common in boys and occurs in all social classes. It is not associated with neurological abnormalities. This includes dyslexia, but a broad-spectrum of problems is recognized.

11.4.2 Developmental coordination disorder

Also known as developmental dyspraxia or clumsy child syndrome, this is another important cause of school difficulties. Apart from difficulty with dressing or physical activities, some children may have great difficulty with writing and drawing. They may be considered wrongly to be stupid or lazy. Incoordination in clumsy children may sometimes represent a mild form of cerebral palsy. Occupational therapy may enable these children to overcome their problems.

11.4.3 Visual impairment

Severe visual impairment is a terrible handicap at any age. Whether it is congenital or originates in early childhood, it presents a serious threat to development and education.

Local authorities keep a register of children with severe visual problems so that the families can be helped and suitable education planned. Experienced home advisers from the local authority or the RNIB (Royal National Institute for the Blind – a charitable organization) visit the family to provide continuing advice and support. They provide practical advice, e.g. 'Wear noisy shoes and give a running commentary about all your household activities so that she can understand and learn about the things she hears, sometimes smells and feels, but never sees'. Most children with visual impairment attend mainstream schools, some of which have specially resourced visual impairment units. Children with more severe visual impairment may attend special schools, some of which are residential. These may teach Braille or use educational material involving large print and type. Schools for the visually impaired are few in number and may be some distance from home.

11.4.4 Squint (strabismus)

Nearly 1 in 15 children have a squint, when they commence school (Figure 11.3). The incidence is even greater in children with brain damage or learning disability. Most squints in children are non-paralytic (concomitant). In non-paralytic squint, there is a normal range of external ocular movements and a constant angle of squint between the two eyes in all directions of gaze. In latent squint, there is extraocular muscle imbalance but the eyes do not deviate most of the time. A latent squint is not visible on inspection and difficult to diagnose. A decrease in visual acuity in one eye can be the cause, so the eyesight should be tested. Paralytic squints, caused by paralysis of one of the external ocular muscles, are unusual in children.

Examination for a squint is a special technique and a favourite of undergraduate examinations (Figure 11.4; see also OSCE station 11.1). Babies sometimes falsely give the impression of having a

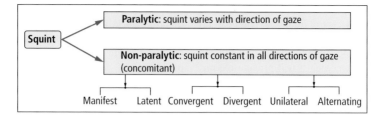

Figure 11.3 Classification of squints. For example, one child may have a manifest, convergent, alternating non-paralytic squint.

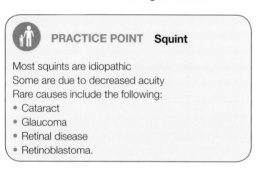

🔑 New-onset paralytic squint may be due to a brain tumour and needs urgent referral.

👥 **PRACTICE POINT   Squint**

Most squints are idiopathic
Some are due to decreased acuity
Rare causes include the following:
- Cataract
- Glaucoma
- Retinal disease
- Retinoblastoma.

---

squint because of a low nasal bridge, epicanthic folds or wide-spaced eyes (*hypertelorism*). This is a *pseudosquint* and is unimportant.

Any child with an untreated squint will suppress vision from the squinting eye in order to avoid blurred images and double vision (Figure 11.5). Unused, the eye can develop permanent *amblyopia* (diminished acuity of central vision). Early treatment before school age should prevent this. If left untreated, vision will be lost in the squinting eye, denying the child binocular vision for life.

Refractive errors are common in children with squints. In many, early use of spectacles is sufficient treatment. Occlusion of the non-squinting eye is unpopular with children. The aim is to force the child to use the squinting eye. Patching or occlusion may be needed for several months. Severe squints may require surgery, if only for cosmetic reasons.

✏️ **TREATMENT   Non-paralytic squint**

- Full ophthalmic examination
- Detection and correction of refractive error
- Patching or occlusion of the squinting eye
- Surgery.

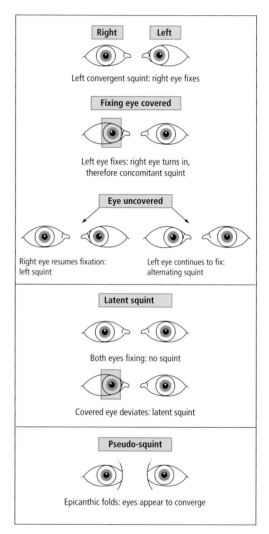

Right   Left

Left convergent squint: right eye fixes

Fixing eye covered

Left eye fixes: right eye turns in, therefore concomitant squint

Eye uncovered

Right eye resumes fixation: left squint

Left eye continues to fix: alternating squint

Latent squint

Both eyes fixing: no squint

Covered eye deviates: latent squint

Pseudo-squint

Epicanthic folds: eyes appear to converge

Figure 11.4 Examination of the eyes for squint. The white dot on the pupil is the reflection of the examiner's torch.

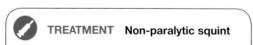

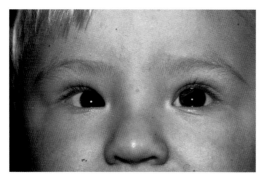

Figure 11.5 This child has a right convergent squint.

11.4.5   Hearing impairment

Hearing exists before birth and can be tested in neonates. They startle to a loud noise or become quiet in response to a quiet voice. In the UK, all newborns go through neonatal screening for sensorineural deafness (Section 10.2.5). At 7–8 months of age, a child's hearing may be tested by distraction testing – does she turn to sound? Pure tone audiometry is not usually possible before 3–4 years.

Congenitally deaf babies are noticed by parents before health professionals. They may have early communication problems or temper tantrums and behavioural problems.

Causes of deafness

Prenatal
- Maternal infection (e.g. rubella)
- Malformation

Perinatal
- Hypoxia
- Prematurity

Postnatal
- Hyperbilirubinaemia
- Infection (meningitis, encephalitis)
- Otitis
- Ototoxic drugs.

Most deaf children have some residual hearing, and so will be helped by a hearing aid, which can be fitted as early as 3 months of age. That is the start of the treatment, not the end. The child requires prolonged exposure to speech and sounds at a level that she can hear with the hearing aid.

Skilled help is needed from a team of otologist, audiologist, hearing aid technician and specially trained teachers. Education for the deaf can be started from early childhood. Most deaf children will enter the partially hearing unit of a nursery school at 3–4 years and then progress to similar units attached to normal schools or to special schools for the deaf.

11.5   Children with special educational needs and disabilities

The normal educational provision of mainstream schools meets the needs of over 80% of children. The rest need something more or something different. In the past, some of these children were labelled according to the nature of their problem (e.g. intellectual disability, physical disability, deaf) and were placed in special schools bearing similar labels. The rest tended to flounder in the bottom layer of mainstream schools, often leaving without any educational qualifications.

More recent policy rests on four principles:

- Early recognition or anticipation of special educational needs
- Detailed assessment through psychological, medical, social, parental and other reports
- Integration into mainstream schools for most, with extra support (the school Special Educational Needs Coordinator – SENCO – is key)
- Special schooling for those who need it.

In the UK, there are two main levels of special support:

1 Extra support within mainstream school environments (e.g. one-to-one help from a teaching assistant, smaller groups, speech and language therapy sessions, support with physical or personal care). This is coordinated by the SENCO. The most common identified need for this level of support is a moderate learning difficulty.
2 Education, health and care plans (EHC) for those with more complex needs (up to age 25). The most common need for children with an EHC is autism spectrum disorder.

11.5.1   Education, health and care (EHC) plans

If a child's needs exceed what can be provided through the first level of support, an EHC plan is created by the local authority, with input and reports from parents and involved professionals in education, health and social care. This has replaced the previous 'Statement of special educational needs', but has a similar function – to define what is needed and how it will be provided. Education for such children may start as early as 2 years and is particularly important for children with visual or hearing impairment, who need to establish good methods of communication with teachers and other children before formal education is possible.

15% of schoolchildren have identified special educational needs.

3% of schoolchildren have EHC plans – half are in mainstream schools.

 Summary

The interaction between health and education is very important for children. Paediatricians, school nurses, audiologists, speech and language therapists and other health professionals work closely with schools and parents to minimize the impact of medical problems. Down syndrome, fragile X and squint often feature in examinations.

 FOR YOUR LOG

- Observe a consultation about learning difficulties.
- Visit a school for children with particular special educational needs, or a specialist inclusion unit within a mainstream school.
- Sit in with an audiologist.

 OSCE TIP

- Examine eyes for squint, vision and eye movements (see OSCE station 11.1).
- General paediatric assessment of learning difficulties.
- Video of child with difficulties.
- Cerebral palsy: need for multidisciplinary approach.

See EMQ 11.1 at the end of the book.

OSCE station 11.1: Examination for squint

Clinical approach:

- Check child understands you and is happy to cooperate
- Note any obviously abnormal neurology

Inspection
- Do eyes look healthy?
- Symmetry
- Normal facies

Acuity
- Simple test that child can see with each eye (with glasses on if worn)
- Does the child wear glasses?

External ocular movements
- Child will follow light, toy or your face
- Test in H pattern

Ophthalmoscopy
- Red reflex
- Are discs and retinae normal? – this can be very difficult, but attempt it

Light reflection
- Hold light near your visual axis (on the end or your nose!)
- When child is fixing on light, is reflection in the middle of both pupils?

Cover test
- Cover fixing eye
- Squinting eye moves and fixes
- Uncover the eye that was covered
- **Either** return to previous eye fixing or previously squinting eye fixes and other eye squints

Billy is 4 years old. Please examine him and tell me if he has a squint

 He wears glasses

Acuity with glasses – identifies little pictures in book – normal

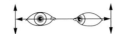

external ocular movements normal

asymmetric light reflection/right eye fixes

 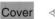 Cover

left eye now fixes (right eye must be squinting)

cover off: left eye returns to squinting + right eye fixes

Billy has a manifest, left, unilateral, convergent squint.

Never forget:

- Say hello and introduce yourself
- General health
- Quickly assess growth, nutrition and development
- Mention the obvious (e.g. drip, leg in plaster)

Look around for:

- Glasses
- Eye patch
- Eye drops

Special points

- Pseudosquints are easily distinguished – the light reflection is symmetrical
- Almost all squints are not due to ocular disease, e.g. retinoblastoma
- Latent squints are too difficult for medical students to find in an examination

SBAs

Q11.1 A neonate is diagnosed clinically with Down syndrome, and blood is sent for karyotype. What further investigation is most important at this point?

a. Chest X-Ray
b. Echocardiogram
c. Full blood count
d. HbA1c
e. Thyroid function tests

Q11.2 A 2-year-old boy has a sudden new onset of a squint in his left eye. He is otherwise well. He has been tilting his head back for a few days. On examination, he has a left 6th nerve palsy.

What is the most appropriate management?

a. Head scan (CT or MRI) urgently
b. Patching of the right eye
c. Reassurance only
d. Referral to ophthalmologist
e. Referral to optician

Q11.3 A 14-year-old boy is seen in a community paediatric clinic with significant learning difficulties. His parents say that his 10-year-old brother is similarly affected. Their mother had some mild learning difficulties as a child. On examination, he has a long thin face, a prominent jaw and unusually large testicles (even allowing for him being post-pubertal).

What test will be most helpful in diagnosis?

a. Genetic testing for Down syndrome
b. Genetic testing for Fragile X
c. IQ test
d. Testosterone level
e. Ultrasound of testicles

For SBA answers, see page 366.

12

Emotional and behavioural problems

Chapter map

Children are unable to express their thoughts and feelings as easily as adults. Emotional disturbances are often expressed either through change in behaviour or through physical symptoms such as aches and pains. The child is part of a family, and problems elsewhere in the family may manifest as emotional and behavioural problems in the child. True psychiatric illness is rare in children. After reviewing attachment and parenting, which are foundational to children's mental health, this chapter discusses types and causes of problems. This provides the basis for management, generally and in regard to specific disorders.

Why emotional and behavioural problems are important

- They affect 5–10% of children in rural areas, 10–20% of children in urban areas.
- Up to one-third of children presenting to their GP or paediatric services have a psychological component to their presentation.

12.1 Attachment

Attachment describes the special relationship that a young child has with his main carers (usually the parents). Young children need to develop at least one secure attachment. A child may have several 'attachment figures', but for young children, the most intense attachment is usually to the mother. Within this attachment relationship is a typical sequence of behaviours that occur again and again:

- The child has a need and expresses it (care-eliciting). For example, a baby cries when he is hungry, or a young child runs to her parent when she is frightened.
- The parent recognizes the need and responds (caregiving). The baby is fed, the young child comforted.
- The child settles, his need met, and his internal balance restored.

Over the early years of life, this repeated sequence builds into the child a model of their world that affects future relationships. With 'good enough' parenting, a secure attachment forms, and the model includes fundamental concepts such as 'I am loveable', 'People will be there for me' and 'People can be trusted'. If caregiving is inconsistent, or even abusive, then the attachment is insecure or ambivalent, and the child's internal model is distorted. Such children find it difficult to form intimate, trusting relationships later on.

Stranger anxiety builds from about 6 months, is maximal at around a year and then slowly recedes as children reach school age (this is why young children need to be examined close to their parents). A child who has not formed secure attachments may be either suspicious and hostile or overly familiar with strangers.

12.1.1   Good enough parenting

No parent is perfect, and most struggle at times with the challenges of bringing up children. Children need a certain level of care to grow and develop both physically and emotionally and to meet their attachment

---

 RESOURCE   **Parenting 'handbooks'**

- *Toddler Taming* by Christopher Green (2006) is full of sensible advice for the first 4 years (e.g. see the chapter on sleep).
- *How to Talk So Kids Will Listen and Listen So Kids Will Talk* by Faber and Mazlish (2013) – does what it says!
- *The Incredible Years* by Webster-Stratton (2006) is the basis for a popular parenting course (see **www.incredibleyears.com**)

---

needs. *Bonding* describes the special relationship that the parents (especially the mother) have with their young child. This bond allows them to love, give to, understand, forgive and cherish their child through good and bad times. Mothers do not necessarily love their baby at first; it may take several weeks. Ideally, parents should be alone with their new baby in quiet, happy and untroubled surroundings, but separation, for example by neonatal illness, does not prevent normal attachment.

12.2   Types of emotional and behavioural problems

Since the causes and management of these problems have much in common, the next part of this chapter will focus on a general approach. Specific problems will then be discussed in more detail.

Good parenting

Positive approach
- Praise > criticism
- Rewards > punishment

Discipline
- Set limits
- Constancy
- Non-victimization
- Non-oppressive

No violence in the home

Opportunities for self-development
- Encourage learning and exploration
- Encourage independence

Stability
- Security within a family home.

Emotional and behavioural problems in children

Infants and pre-school children	Older children	
Behavioural	*Behavioural*	*Stress-related*
Tantrums	Defiant	Headaches
Sleep problems	Impulsive	Abdominal
Feeding difficulties	Attention deficit	pains
Crying babies	Lying	Vomiting
Breath-holding	Stealing	Wetting
attacks	Truancy	Soiling
	Tics	

12.3 Causes of emotional and behavioural problems

There are many factors which lead to these problems (Figure 12.1). Children's symptoms vary greatly, and there is often no clear relationship between particular behavioural problems and specific causes. Most often it is to do with the child's interactions or relationships with important people around them. Many problems are exaggerations of normal behaviour, unintentionally maintained through the way they are being handled, especially if there are inconsistencies between parents.

12.3.1 Child factors

The form that an emotional disturbance takes will depend in part upon the cause and in part upon the child's personality and the family patterns of response to stress. Some children are of a buoyant temperament and can ride almost any crisis; others are sensitive to emotional disturbances. The way parents respond to the problem may inadvertently exacerbate or perpetuate these problems. Stress may present as headache, tempers or abdominal pain in different children. The toddler who feels challenged by the arrival of a new baby may resort to infantile behaviour.

12.3.2 Family factors

12.3.2.1 Acute separation and change

The death of a parent or of a much-loved grandparent, emergency admission to hospital or moving house are examples of acute separations. These are most upsetting to young children around 2–4 years old who are conscious of the separation but unable to understand the reason.

12.3.2.2 Parental discord and separation

All children are conscious of the relationship between their parents and will be aware of any deterioration. Parents who attempt to get their children to take sides during conflict make this an even more difficult experience.

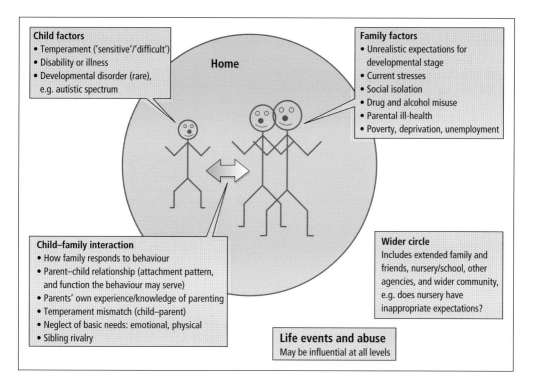

Child factors
- Temperament ('sensitive'/'difficult')
- Disability or illness
- Developmental disorder (rare), e.g. autistic spectrum

Home

Family factors
- Unrealistic expectations for developmental stage
- Current stresses
- Social isolation
- Drug and alcohol misuse
- Parental ill-health
- Poverty, deprivation, unemployment

Child–family interaction
- How family responds to behaviour
- Parent–child relationship (attachment pattern, and function the behaviour may serve)
- Parents' own experience/knowledge of parenting
- Temperament mismatch (child–parent)
- Neglect of basic needs: emotional, physical
- Sibling rivalry

Wider circle
Includes extended family and friends, nursery/school, other agencies, and wider community, e.g. does nursery have inappropriate expectations?

Life events and abuse
May be influential at all levels

Figure 12.1 Possible sources of child behaviour problems.

RESOURCE   Children and parental divorce or separation

Health professionals are sometimes asked for advice about helping children through divorce or separation. Here are some useful starting points:
- **www.rcpsych.ac.uk** has a useful factsheet (search for 'divorce' on their site) as part of their excellent 'Mental Health and Growing Up' series.
- **www.raisingchildren.net.au** is an Australian site – search there for 'Me and my changing family', an online book, which offers tips on building healthy relationships after separation. A few items are specific to Australia.

12.3.3   Child–family interaction

12.3.3.1   Inconsistent handling

If a child is permitted something by one parent that is denied by the other, or punished on one occasion and ignored on another, this is likely to lead to behavioural problems. The intelligent child is quick to play off one adult against another, or to achieve her own ends by alarming or distressing the adults around her.

12.3.3.2   Lack of parental time

All children need regular positive attention, especially from their parents. When this is lacking, then the negative attention given for bad behaviour can become enough of a reward to reinforce the behaviour. This can lead to a vicious cycle of more negative attention (e.g. telling off, punishing) leading to worsening behaviour.

12.3.3.3   Sibling rivalry

Most toddlers, and especially first-borns, delight in the new baby, but may resent the time that their mother devotes to it. Aggression is likely to be directed against the mother rather than against the baby. When the new baby is old enough to be mobile and to interfere with the elder sibling's activities, jealousy will become more obvious. At school age, constant comparisons between siblings with different capabilities and interests can devastate the less clever or the clumsy.

12.3.3.4   Great expectations

Parents naturally want their child to do well, but may form an unrealistic idea of her capabilities or set their hearts on a career which she could never achieve. Although many a child 'could do better if she tried', not everyone is destined for an honours degree. If parents constantly nag when she is doing her best,

psychological difficulties may follow. Somatization is common (e.g. abdominal pains).

12.3.4   Wider circle

Do not forget to explore the child's life outside the immediate family. Remember school, nursery and the extended family. All of these may have an impact and offer you insight into problems that are occurring. Although most schools try to minimize bullying, it is still a common and important cause of behavioural problems. Contact with the school or nursery (with the parents' permission) is often helpful.

12.3.5   Life events and abuse

Sometimes a child is witness to, or involved in, an acutely distressing situation – a road accident, sudden death or sexual abuse. This may lead to a variety of symptoms such as disturbed behaviour (e.g. night terrors), or to acute physical symptoms (e.g. overbreathing). An event like this may have severe long-term effects.

12.4   Management

12.4.1   General approach to the management of behavioural problems

Most behavioural problems in young children respond to a calm and consistent approach that emphasizes the positive. Identify and build on the strengths of the child and family. Encourage parents to work together, and to use distraction and/or change of activity when the problem behaviour is first noticed. Simple explanation helps parents realize that these problems are extremely common and part of normal experience. They do not need to feel there is something fundamentally 'wrong' or 'bad' about themselves or their child.

12.4.1.1   Strategies

- Positive reinforcement:
  - Reward desired behaviours with warmth, praise and small tokens (e.g. stars on a star chart)
  - Ignore undesired behaviours
- Time out:
  - Child removed from the situation for 3 min
  - Breaks a negative cycle
  - Calms things

- Promote positive parent–child times:
  - Good times when contentious issues are set aside
  - Affirmation of the child through gesture (e.g. cuddles)
  - Activities enjoyed together (e.g. trips, crafts)
- Set and apply clear limits, where consequences of behaviours are as follows:
  - Clearly understood
  - Applied consistently, quickly and without argument
  - Appropriate in magnitude.

 PRACTICE POINT Star charts

Especially, useful in early school-age children based on operant conditioning – reinforcing the desired behaviour and ignoring (and thus 'extinguishing') the unwanted behaviour the giving of stars should be:

- Achievable – otherwise lack of stars will demoralize
- Consistent – all carers do the same
- Immediate – the younger the child, the more quickly the star should be given
- Clear – child and parents are clear what the star is for
- Contingent – only give the star for the identified behaviour.

12.4.2 General approach to the management of stress-related (psychosomatic) symptoms

A large part of clinical practice involves children (and adults) with pains and other symptoms for which no satisfactory cause can be found. Deciding whether the symptoms are secondary to stress can be difficult. History, examination and growth monitoring will usually exclude serious disease. It is rarely helpful to label a pain as psychogenic, which may be interpreted as imagined or fabricated.

Adopt a comprehensive approach and accept that all symptoms result from interaction of body and mind, and that expression of physical disorder or good health is modified not just by physical factors, but also by intellectual, emotional and social factors.

12.4.2.1 Stress-related symptoms and tests

Avoid tests if possible. If tests are necessary, it is better to say:

'I think your symptoms are stress-related but I want to do some tests to make sure' rather than:

'I will do some tests to exclude physical problems. If they are negative, it must be stress-related' (you will end up running out of tests!).

After listening to the history, there are two useful questions, 'What sort of a boy is he?' Children with stress symptoms are more often described as nervous, worriers, perfectionists or solitary than as placid, happy-go-lucky or gregarious. 'Who does he take after?' may elicit a rueful smile and the admission that one or both parents are similar. This helps understanding. Examination reveals no abnormal signs.

Stress symptoms do not just disappear. It is helpful to reassure that there is no organic disease. Explain the nature of the symptoms and encourage the family not to pay undue attention to them. Make it clear that you understand that the pains are real and not imaginary. Every effort should be made to identify and address stresses. Health visitors and teachers can be helpful. A careful history and examination coupled with firm reassurance is important and may be all that is needed.

Diaries – ABC approach

- A simple diary kept by parents between appointments often clarifies the problem
- Recording informed by the 'ABC approach' may lead to a solution in its own right, as parents gain a greater understanding
- For several episodes ask parents to note: **A**ntecedents (trigger/s); nature of the **B**ehaviour; the immediate **C**onsequences for the child (as well as what conclusions he/she makes about them)

12.5 Specific disorders

Some of the following disorders are covered in more detail elsewhere in this book. Follow the cross-references for more details.

12.5.1 Stress-related symptoms

12.5.1.1 Recurrent abdominal pain

Abdominal pain is a common childhood symptom, and the commonest causes are constipation and stress-related symptoms (of which some may be due to irritable bowel syndrome, non-ulcer dyspepsia and abdominal migraine) (Section 22.1.2).

12.5.1.2 Stress headaches

Stress headaches are usually frontal. In some cases, headache is the family stress symptom (Section 18.9).

12.5.1.3 Tics

These repetitive involuntary movements are usually worse with stress. A low key reassuring approach is best (Section 18.9).

12.5.1.4 Vomiting

Vomiting is intimately connected with the emotions ('I'm sick of it all') but is less common than pain as a stress symptom. It occurs at a younger age than recurrent pains (Section 22.1.1).

12.5.1.5 Wetting problems

Both day- and night-time wetting may occur due to organic factors such as detrusor instability or urinary tract infection, but may be triggered or worsened by stress (Section 23.6).

12.5.2 Behavioural and sleep-related

12.5.2.1 Disturbance of bowel habit

Potty training may be started any time in the first 2 years, and a few parents choose to defer it for longer. If started very young, it is the parents who are training themselves to put a pot under the baby when he is going to pass faeces or urine, most commonly after a feed. This helps to establish a conditioned reflex, reinforced by praise when something arrives in the pot but not by punishing the reverse. Toddlers should not be left sitting on their pots for long periods, nor should potty training be obsessional or coercive ('You can't until. . .'). Faulty bowel training predisposes towards constipation, which may become lifelong.

Bowel disturbances

- Chronic constipation, which may be complicated by faecal soiling (Section 22.1.5)
- Faecal incontinence resulting from neurological disorders
- Encopresis: deliberate defaecation in inappropriate places. Usually indicates emotional distress
- Toddler diarrhoea (Section 22.1.4).

12.5.2.2 Sleep difficulties

Sleepless children demoralize parents. Young children are demanding by day, but parents survive if they can enjoy peaceful nights. Sleeplessness may begin for a good reason, but persist as a bad habit. Children differ in their personalities from birth.

Young infants sleep most of the time, and crying usually indicates hunger, thirst, cold or pain. Anxiety or depression in the family may make things worse. The most difficult sleep problems are usually seen in toddlers. Some do not settle down when put to bed: others sleep for a few hours and are then full of activity when the rest of the household is sound asleep. By the time advice is sought, these habits have usually persisted for a long time and parents have tried both protracted and complicated bedtime routines, and the almost irreversible step of admitting the child to the parental bed. It is noticeable that whilst the parents often look worn out, the offending child has boundless energy.

Sleep disorders may date from an illness or upset in which a few broken nights were to be expected, but has been protracted by over-solicitous attention. Another common cause is putting the child to bed too early or at no fixed time.

Management of sleep problems

- Returning to sleep from the normal transient awakenings that occur through the night is a learned behaviour. If a child associates the process of going to sleep with a factor that is not there later in the night (e.g. bottle, dummy, sleeping next to parent) they are more likely to have disturbed sleep ('sleep-association disorder').
- Avoid or reduce daytime naps.
- Establish a calm bedtime routine.
- When the child wakes and cries leave him to cry for a pre-planned time, e.g. 2–5 min, then settle with as little physical contact as possible (neither kisses nor recriminations) and leave again. Continue to check on the crying child after repeating the same time delay.

- Avoid sedative medication. Behavioural techniques are far more likely to achieve a long-term solution.

12.5.2.3 Nightmares

Bad dreams are common at all ages. Parents, having experienced them themselves, are not usually very worried by them. They know that nightmares occur in normal people and that they do not mean major emotional upset. Measures such as leaving the bedroom door open, or a light on, may comfort the child who is frightened of going to bed. Nightmares occur during rapid eye movement (REM) sleep and are the culmination of a frightening dream adventure, the details of which the child can remember immediately afterwards.

12.5.2.4 Night terrors

Night terrors are not common, but are most alarming. They occur mainly in the first hour or two of sleep in children between 2 and 8 years. The child shrieks, sits up and stares wide-eyed and terrified as if being attacked by something only he can see. He may stumble out of bed and seem oblivious to the parents' soothing words. However, within a few minutes he will be sound asleep again and will remember nothing in the morning. Night terrors occur during non-REM sleep and occur abruptly (not as the result of a dream sequence). They are accompanied by an alarming rise of the pulse and violent respirations which may at times make the parents or doctor suspect an epileptic fit. The parents can be reassured that night terrors do not indicate serious psychological abnormality and that the child will outgrow them. Gently calming the child back to sleep is all that is needed. If they occur at a regular time of night, the child can be woken just before this.

12.5.2.5 Sleepwalking

This may occur independently or as an extension of night terrors, though the sleepwalker tends to be slightly older (e.g. 6–12 years). The child gets out of bed and may walk around the house or even into the street. Although difficult to awaken, he can be guided back to bed. Regardless of that, he will usually find his own way back to bed and to sleep.

Neither sleepwalking nor night terrors should be considered as evidence of major emotional disturbance. Both conditions tend to be familial and to disappear before adolescence.

12.5.2.6 Crying babies

All normal babies cry. Excessive crying, especially at night, exhausts parents and is a known risk factor for physical abuse. Pain (e.g. earache) may be responsible for short-term crying. Persistent crying more often reflects household tensions. Mothers who seek advice about excessive crying may be afraid that they or their husbands will lose their tempers and damage the baby. The problem may sound trivial to a busy doctor but must *always* be taken seriously. The health visitor can often help.

12.5.2.7 Breath-holding attacks

Sometimes mistaken for seizures, but always triggered by some event or upset (Section 18.3, p. 192).

12.5.2.8 Tantrums

Tantrums are normal to toddlerhood. Give reassurance, telling parents how common tantrums are and show empathy. Some tantrums are promoted by boredom, frustration, inconsistent handling and repeated unnecessary thwarting of activities which can be preventable. Explanation of normal development and the limits of children's abilities and understanding can prepare parents for the inevitable tantrum and need for limit setting. Bad or negative attention is still more rewarding than no attention. Tantrums are best managed by distracting the child away from the tantrum to another activity. Avoid giving rewarding attention to the tantrum. Everybody who looks after the child must handle the tantrums in the same way.

12.5.2.9 Feeding difficulties in the young child (Table 12.1)

- Weigh and measure accurately.
- Base all interventions on a food diary.

12.5.3 Severe behavioural disorders

Anorexia nervosa is covered in Section 17.4.2.

12.5.3.1 Autism spectrum disorder (ASD)

The term 'spectrum' is used because children with this pervasive developmental disorder share similar characteristics that shade into each other (Figure 12.2). At their heart is an inability to read the

Table 12.1 **Common problems with feeding**	
Problem	**Solution**
Child easily distracted by TV or runs round room at mealtimes.	Turn off TV: mealtime must be the focus and ideally family members all eat together with child in high or other safe chair and table.
Children change their mind about what they are willing to eat.	Either make only one meal for all the family, or offer child a choice of two things and, if appropriate, allow child to help in preparation.
Child very slow eater or picks at food.	If weight satisfactory, reassure parent–child will not starve. Don't hurry child or force-feed. Present food for an agreed fixed period of time and then remove it.
Too much fluid, either milk almost entirely in place of food or excessive drinking of fruit juice or pop.	Give drinks and snacks after, not before, meals.

minds of others. The normal processing of verbal and non-verbal cues and signals is impaired so that the child cannot 'think himself into someone else's shoes': he cannot imagine what someone else is thinking or feeling. Instead, the brain seems configured to process information about systems and things, to varying degrees of ability. This produces problems in communication, behaviour and social interaction (Figure 12.2). The relative level of difficulty and ability in each area determines the child's position on the spectrum, and there are formal scoring tools to help with this. A long list of other paediatric disorders has been associated with the autism spectrum, so it is important to complete a detailed evaluation.

PRACTICE POINT

Consider autism spectrum disorder in a child who is not speaking – especially if they are silent and do not communicate non-verbally (e.g. eye contact and pointing).

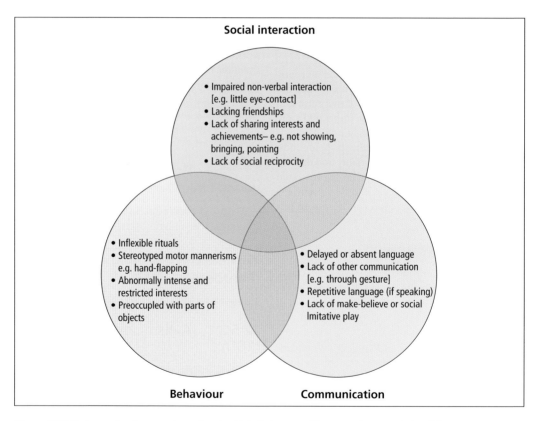

Figure 12.2 Features of autism spectrum disorder. Note that some of these can be normal at certain ages, so assessment should take account of developmental stage. Some features in each area are needed to make a diagnosis.

About 0.5% of children are thought to be on the autism spectrum. Sometimes the onset of symptoms is very early; a mother may say, 'As a baby he would never let me cuddle him'. Usually they present in the second or third year of life with language or behaviour problems. Autism spectrum disorder is a lifelong condition and can be very disabling. Early detection and skilled educational and behavioural intervention by a multi-disciplinary team are recommended. Some autistic behaviour is not uncommon amongst children with other learning disorders. There is no evidence linking autism to MMR immunization (Section 15.2).

 TREATMENT **Management**

- Foster developmental progress
- Promote learning
- Reduce stereotyped behaviours
- Eliminate maladaptive behaviour
- Alleviate family distress – family support and education

Some children with autism spectrum disorder have less severe behavioural features, and normal intelligence, and may merely appear odd or eccentric. They often have difficulties at school. The distress can be greater than with 'classic' autism because the child has greater insight.

12.5.3.2 Attention-deficit and hyperactivity disorder (ADHD)

Children vary greatly in the extent of their activity and concentration, and it is impossible to define the limit between physiological and pathological degrees of overactivity. Many normal children are 'always on the go', 'never still' and need relatively few hours of sleep. Beyond this is the Attention-deficit and hyperactivity disorder (ADHD) syndrome in which these features

ADHD syndrome

- Inattention
  - Changes activity frequently
  - Will not persist with tasks
  - Short attention span
- Hyperactivity
  - Fidgetiness
  - Restlessness
- Impulsiveness
  - Impetuous erratic behaviour
  - Frequent accidents
  - Thoughtless rule breaking.

interfere with learning or development. In children of school age, this presents a grave educational problem.

ADHD is more common in boys and in children with evidence of brain damage, which further complicates their education. Behaviour modification therapy can help. For some, methylphenidate may have a quietening effect, but drug therapy may be difficult to stop. In some children, hyperactivity is caused or aggravated by particular foods or (more often) colourings. A properly supervised exclusion diet is worth trying: any improvement in behaviour will be evident within a few days.

 # Summary

Most emotional and behavioural problems are exaggerations of normal behaviour, unintentionally maintained through the way they are being handled. Assessment should include the context and the many potential sources of behaviour problems. Consider several appointments, use of diaries and charts, and wide consultation. Management involves addressing underlying problems where possible, but specific useful techniques include explanation, positive reinforcement, avoiding reward of undesired behaviours, time out, promoting positive family times and use of clear limits.

 FOR YOUR LOG

- Observe the use of star charts and symptom diaries in outpatient clinics.
- Observe attachment behaviour in children on the wards and in clinics.
- Discuss some of the common behaviour problems of young children with parents.

 OSCE TIP

- Stress-related conditions (e.g. pain, headache) (see OSCE station 12.1).
- Enuresis: explain to parent, enuresis alarm.
- Constipation and soiling: history, explanation.
- Video of attention-deficit disorder.

See Chapter 12 EMQs: 'Treatment of continence problems in children', 'Headache' and 'Abdominal pain' in the EMQ section at the end of the book.

References

Faber, A. and Mazlish, E. (2013). *How To Talk So Kids Will Listen and Listen So Kids Will Talk*. London: Piccadilly Press.

Green, C. (2006). *New Toddler Taming. A Parents' Guide to the First Four Years*. London: Vermilion.

Webster-Stratton, C. (2006). *The Incredible Years: A Guide for Parents of Children 2–8 Years Old*. Seattle, USA: The Incredible Years, Inc.

OSCE station 12.1: History-taking – pain

Clinical approach:
- Begin with open questions (e.g. could you tell me what worries you?)
- Then focus to more specific questions

Pain
- Nature
- Site
- First and last occurrence
- Duration of each episode
- Frequency
- Length of history
  ◦ Severity
  ◦ How bad is it?
  ◦ Can parents tell pain is present?
  ◦ Does it stop him playing/ going back to school?
- Timing
  ◦ Day/night, etc.
  ◦ School days/holidays
- Modifying factors
  ◦ Stress
  ◦ Medicines
  ◦ Food/starvation

Associated symptoms
- Vomiting
- Diarrhoea/constipation
- Enuresis/dysuria
- Headache

Gary is 11 years old. His mother is worried about his abdominal pain. He has not been at school for 4 weeks. Please take a brief history

- Mother's biggest worry: Gary is missing time at his new school

- Central ache
- Most of each day
- Not at night
- Better at weekends
- Appetite good
- Sleeping well
- No other symptoms

- Gary's mother is clearly very anxious
- Gary is not present. He spends most of his time watching TV
- No other significant history

Gary has stress-related abdominal pain. It may have been precipitated by the move to a new school. The mother is usually a member of staff who has been given a history

Never forget:
- Say hello and introduce yourself
- Tell the parent(s) and child what you aim to do
- General health – is the child ill?
- Ask, is there anything else you think I should know?

If asked or time permits:
- Full history
- Do not forget
  ◦ Birth history
  ◦ Development
  ◦ Immunizations
  ◦ Family/social history

Look around for:
- Family interaction
- Parental anxiety
- Evidence of care or neglect

Special points
- If exact answer not known (e.g. how long?) ask for approximate answer
- Ask if problem is getting better, getting worse, or staying the same
- What do the parents think about the cause of the pain?
- Does severity of pain match impact on the child's life (e.g. time off school?)

SBAs

Q12.1 A 5 year old has a history of screaming inconsolably shortly after falling asleep on some nights and does not appear to respond to their parents comforting. They then settle and fall back asleep.

What is the most likely cause?

a.   Benign Rolandic Epilepsy
b.   Breath-holding attacks
c.   Nightmares
d.   Night terrors
e.   Reflex anoxic seizures

Q12.2 There are concerns that a 7-year-old boy is not paying attention is school, is easily distracted and is not completing tasks. They fidget often, can't sit still in class and have impetuous behaviour.

What diagnosis would fit with this presentation?

a.   Absence seizures
b.   Anxiety
c.   Attention-deficit hyperactivity disorder
d.   Autism spectrum disorder

For SBA answers, see page 367.

13

Nutrition

Chapter map

Infant and child nutrition is the foundation stone of healthy development. Worldwide, the most important problem is malnutrition. In industrialized societies, the main problem is the increase in childhood obesity. In clinical practice, nutritional care is central to the management of all chronic diseases.

Nutrition is particularly important in the first year of life, when the infant is entirely dependent on his carers to feed him. Babies treble their birthweight in the first year of life and to treble it again takes 10 years. In fact, 65% of total postnatal brain growth takes place in the first year of life. Malnutrition may permanently disrupt physical and mental development.

PRACTICE POINT

Parents are often concerned about feeding, odd stools and small vomits. The first step is to plot the infant's weight on a growth chart. Normal growth is greatly reassuring.

Poor foetal nutrition and then rapid weight gain in the first years greatly increases risk of adult diabetes and cardiovascular disease: an example of nutritional programming.

13.1 Infant nutrition

Average requirements in infancy

Water   150 mL/kg/day

Calories   110 kcal/kg/day

13.1.1 Milk

Milk is a rich source of energy, proteins and minerals. It is the sole source of nutrition for the first months and provides an essential part of energy, protein and calcium intake in preschool children. Cow's milk has a high mineral content and osmolality. Infant formula feeds are modified to be more like breast milk.

Unmodified cow's milk should not be given in the first year: breast or formula feeding is recommended

immunodeficiency virus (HIV) infection in developed countries (but not in the developing world, where the benefits still outweigh the small risk). 'Breast milk jaundice' is not a reason to stop (Section 9.4.2, p. 91).

13.1.3 Bottle feeding

Formula feeds are available in two forms: whey dominant (60% whey) like breast milk and casein dominant (30% whey). The former is more akin to breast milk and should be first choice. Each of the four UK milk manufacturers makes two milks so that a mother can change milks without changing company. There are no major advantages to different manufacturers' milks, and parents should be dissuaded from constantly changing milk. Follow-on formula should not be used before 6 months. Their use after that age is popular but not necessary. Attention to detail in making up the feed is essential. Extra scoops, heaped scoops, packed scoops or additional cereal should be avoided. They add calories which encourage obesity, and extra solutes which cause thirst, irritability and hypernatraemia. It is conventional to warm feeds to approximately body temperature, but this is not always needed.

> **Bottle feeding requirements**
>
> **Meticulous care in hygiene**
> **Sterilizing bottles**
> **Correct feed reconstitution for a 4-oz bottle (110 mL)**
> - Take 4 oz of cooled boiled tap water
> - Fill scoop without compressing powder
> - Scrape scoop level with clean knife
> - Add four scoops of powder
> - Dissolve, allow to cool to about 37 °C
> - May be refrigerated
> - Only rewarm once.

> **PRACTICE POINT**
>
> Soya-based formulae do not prevent food allergy or atopic disease. Soya formulae should not be used under 6 months.

Feeds should be given either 4 hourly or on demand. The newborn baby will require feeding round the clock, but within a few weeks will drop the night feed. As long as a night feed is demanded, it should be given. Leaving the baby to cry is pointless and unkind.

13.1.4 Mixed feeding

The term *weaning* is variously used to mean taking the baby off the breast or introducing solid foods (Figure 13.3). A full-term baby receiving milk will not develop any nutritional deficiency within 6 months of birth. The WHO and UK advice is that solids should be given at 6 months, although in practice a majority of European infants receive solids from 4 months onwards. Solids before 3 months are ill-advised. Early weaning is linked to later obesity.

- Use pureed fruit, vegetable and rice as first foods.
- Ensure an adequate introduction of food containing protein and iron.
- Introduce one new food at a time in small quantities.
- Increase solids in diet as chewing begins around 6 months.
- The average 1-year-old will be having three main meals a day, with a small drink or snack mid-morning, mid-afternoon and at bedtime. Milk intake 20–30 oz/day (600–900 mL).

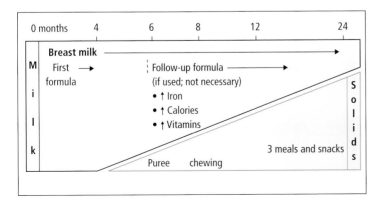

Figure 13.3 Weaning.

PRACTICE POINT

Many parents (and doctors) still use ounces:
1 fluid ounce = 28 mL
1 pint = 560 mL.

13.1.5 Iron and vitamin supplements

In the UK, vitamin A, C and D supplements are recommended for all children aged 6 months to 5 years. In low-income and at-risk groups, these are available via the 'Healthy Start' programme. Supplements may be made available to the wider population (already happening in some countries), because targeted provision is logistically difficult, and there is increasing concern about widespread subclinical vitamin D deficiency. Clinical vitamin deficiency states are rare. Some parents may choose to give a children's multivitamin supplement, and this is safe.

Folic acid is provided by leaf vegetables and fruits. Vitamin D may be derived from cholesterol through the action of sunlight. It is contained in oily (non-white) fish, liver and margarines. An increasing proportion of vitamin intake comes from 'fortified' foods: formula milk, bread, breakfast cereals and fruit-flavoured drinks. In prematurity, chronic illness or poor diet, vitamin supplements are important.

Iron-deficiency anaemia occurs in around 15–25% of toddlers in areas of socioeconomic deprivation. It can be prevented with use of iron-enriched formula.

13.2 Nutrition of toddlers and school children

Changing social patterns in industrialized countries have had profound influences, not necessarily beneficial, on the nutrition of children. A tradition of home cooking, and indeed home growing of vegetables, has given place to supermarket shopping, fast and convenience foods and takeaway meals. This pattern is now established across the socioeconomic groups and persists even in the areas or times of deprivation.

Recent concerns about food additives (artificial flavourings, colourings, sweeteners, preservative), food provenance and food allergies have turned some families towards 'natural' food and a return to home cooking.

The chief nutritional requirements of children are protein for building new tissue as they grow, and sufficient fat and carbohydrate to meet their substantial energy needs. Protein requirements (milk, egg, fish, meat, cereals and pulses) are about 1–1.5 g/kg/day. Energy requirements are high compared with most adults, who need less than a third of a child's requirements/kg.

The dietary basis of obesity, dental caries and much constipation in childhood is well accepted. Refined sugar should be eaten in moderation and sticky sweets preferably not at all (or at least not continuously!). An excess of fried foods (e.g. hamburgers and french fries) encourages obesity, and public opinion has now forced recognition of this in fast-food outlets. Fibre helps prevent constipation. Most fizzy drinks ('pop') have little or no nutritional value and help to rot teeth. Milk is highly nutritious (400 kcal/pint) but an excessive intake can contribute to obesity.

Energy requirements (kcal/kg/day)	
Maintenance	80
Growth	5
Physical activity	25
Total	110

13.3 Feeding problems

PRACTICE POINT

Beware of modifying a young child's diet without dietetic help!

13.3.1 Early problems

Difficulties with feeding are common and may cause great anxiety. Feeding problems may present with vomiting, disturbed bowel habit, unsatisfactory weight gain or crying. Most difficulties arise from one or more of three factors:

1 *Quantity* of food. Both underfeeding and overfeeding may lead to vomiting and crying. In the first, weight gain is consistently poor. An overfed baby gains weight excessively to begin with, but may later lose. Overfeeding is more common in bottle-fed babies, partly because they are often fed as much as they can take, partly because food has a sedative effect, and partly because of the mistaken belief that the biggest babies are the best.

PRACTICE POINT

Luke is 8 days old and is at home. He is breastfeeding. He is unwell, quiet and lethargic. On examination, he has lost 14% of his birthweight, but does not look clinically dehydrated. Investigations show a high serum sodium (154 mmol/L), and he is quite jaundiced.

Luke has hypernatraemic dehydration which is often difficult to detect because the clinical signs of dehydration may not be present. The problem is lactation failure, and the clue is his weight loss. After slow rehydration and breastfeeding support, lactation was established and he thrived well.

2 *Kind* of food. Early mixed feeding may lead to vomiting, diarrhoea and crying. A return to a milk diet will allow recovery, followed by cautious reintroduction of solids. Changing from one milk to another rarely achieves anything.

3 Feeding *technique*. The mother who wishes to breastfeed should be given help, support and practical advice. This comes from experienced professionals or groups such as the National Childbirth Trust (NCT: www.nctpregnancyandbabycare.com). Difficulties with bottle feeding can only be recognized by watching the baby feeding. The baby may not be held comfortably; the bottle may be held at the wrong angle; the hole in the teat may be too small or too big; the milk may have been wrongly prepared. Instruction and advice provide the remedy.

PRACTICE POINT
Always check growth

You can quickly estimate expected weight: birthweight is regained after 10 days (normal loss is 5–7% of birthweight, max 10%). Then, babies gain 200 g/week (an ounce a day).

13.3.2 Infantile colic

Infantile colic, or evening colic, is a common problem arising in early life. It is usually better by 4 months. An otherwise placid baby devotes one part of the day, most commonly between the 6 p.m. and 10 p.m. feeds, to incessant crying. He may stop when picked up, but certainly cries again if put down. Attention to feeds, warmth, wet nappies, etc. does not help. The cause is unknown. First reassure and monitor growth. Anti-bubbling agents (Infacol) may be helpful. In severe colic, some infants respond to a diet free of cow's milk with a formula feed containing hydrolysed proteins.

13.3.3 Sucking and feeding

Most babies take a feed in 20–30 min. Some drain a bottle in 5–10 min and may then have filled their stomachs. Infants may find comfort in non-nutritive sucking on a thumb or a dummy, but the latter should be avoided in the first few weeks while breastfeeding is being established.

From 6 months, an increasing diversity of foods and textures should be tried, and the child allowed to learn the joy of eating – even if this is not the tidiest of processes. Major conflict is best avoided. There is a delicate distinction between encouraging the conservative child to try something new, and coercing the reluctant child to eat 'what is good for him'. Parents are best advised to back off from conflict and to developing good mealtime rituals. It is helpful to note that no normal child with access to food will starve; that children of some ages are dominated by the need for food, but at other ages it may be a low priority; that wise parents do not start battles with their children that they are bound to lose; and that a parent will often achieve most by doing least.

13.4 Defective nutrition

13.4.1 Obesity

Obesity in childhood is a common and important problem – important to the child, the family and public health. The tendency to excessive weight gain may appear in infancy, toddlerhood or during school years. Obese children often come from overweight families and are likely to become obese as adults. The proportion of the population overweight or obese rises with age: 1/5 of 4- to 5-year-olds, 1/3rd of 10- to

11-year-olds and 60% of adults in England. The essential problem is energy intake exceeding energy needs. Deficiency of leptin, which normally signals calorie sufficiency, may be important but, in the vast majority of obese children, no cause is found. Obese children are nearly always tall for their age.

> **PRACTICE POINT**
>
> Obesity combined with short stature suggests an underlying pathology, such as endocrine disease and merits investigations.

Co-morbidities associated with obesity in childhood

- Psychological: poor self-esteem
- Obstructive sleep apnoea
- Slipped upper femoral epiphysis
- Type 2 diabetes
- Hypertension
- Abnormal blood lipids
- Non-alcoholic fatty liver disease
- Polycystic ovarian syndrome

Obesity may limit exercise tolerance. The dominant symptoms in childhood are psychological. The overweight or obese child may be teased and ostracized, losing self-esteem. In boys, the disappearance of the penis into a pad of suprapubic fat may lead to a mistaken diagnosis of hypogonadism.

A body mass index (BMI) (Section 3.2.4, p. 35) (kg/m²) over the 98th centile is diagnostic. In the obese child, weight reduction is advisable but impossible to procure without the enthusiastic collaboration of the child and their family.

13.4.2   Malnutrition

Marasmus is due to energy (calorie) and protein starvation.
Kwashiorkor is the result of protein malnutrition.

13.4.2.1   Marasmus

Nutritional deficiency ranges from starvation to lack of specific nutrients: in Europe, starvation is seen in children who have been grossly neglected, but in parts of the world afflicted by poverty, famine or war, *infantile marasmus* is all too common. Breastfeeding continues for about 2 years, but when supply of breast milk is inadequate, starvation ensues. The infant with marasmus is prey to intercurrent infection, and mortality is high. There is also evidence that starvation in the first year of life, even if subsequently corrected, may cause permanent mental handicap.

13.4.2.2   Kwashiorkor

This is seen in the same parts of the world as marasmus but in older children, usually 2–4 years old. At this age, the next baby often displaces the older sibling from the breast. Milk is replaced by a low protein, starch (rice or maize)-based diet. The child is listless, the face, limbs and abdomen swell, the hair is sparse, dry and depigmented, and there are areas of hyperpigmentation ('black enamel paint') especially on the legs. Diarrhoea is sometimes a feature.

13.4.2.3   Vitamin deficiencies

Worldwide, vitamin deficiencies remain an appalling problem for children. Vitamin A deficiency is the single most important cause of childhood blindness worldwide. Initial loss of dark adaptation is followed by corneal disease (xerophthalmia), which may lead to irreversible corneal perforation. An estimated 250 000 young children each year suffer from xerophthalmia, and nearly 10 million suffer from lesser degrees of deficiency. Supplementation is cheap, protective and reduces infection.

Some European families adopt bizarre diets for their own reasons, and growing children fed on such diets may be malnourished. In contrast, children on a vegetarian diet are usually healthy (and most unlikely to be obese). Specific nutritional deficiencies such as scurvy (vitamin C deficiency with bleeding into gums and subperiosteum) are very rare in otherwise healthy children.

13.4.2.4   Rickets

Nutritional rickets results from dietary deficiency of vitamin D coupled with inadequate exposure to sunlight (Figure 13.4). It presents at times of active growth – in the preschool years of life and at puberty. It is more common in Asian children in the UK because the traditional diet is poor in calcium and they receive little sunlight on their skin.

Deficiency of calcium, phosphorus or vitamin D interferes with bone maturation, leading to a

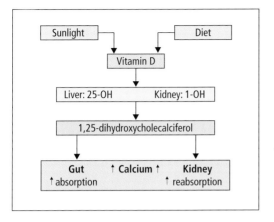

Figure 13.4 Vitamin D metabolism.

build-up of osteoid tissue. Thickening of the metaphyses where active growth is most rapid is seen at the wrists, ankles and costochondral junctions ('rickety rosary') (Figure 13.5). Toddlers develop bow legs: older children become knock-kneed. There is hypotonia. In children with malabsorption, rickets declares itself when growth is rapid because it is a disease of growing bones. Serum calcium is normal or reduced, and the alkaline phosphatase is raised. Some present with hypocalcaemic fits. Adequate vitamin D intake prevents rickets.

All baby milk foods and most cereals have vitamin D added. Treatment of rickets requires dietary education and supplementary vitamin D.

Renal rickets has two main origins:

- *Glomerular* disease in chronic renal failure leads to failure of hydroxylation of vitamin D in the kidney to the active form (1,25-dihydroxycholecalciferol).
- *Tubular* renal rickets. Failure of normal tubular reabsorption of phosphate occurs (e.g. vitamin D-resistant rickets).

13.5   Nutrition in chronic disease

In many chronic diseases of childhood, nutritional care is an essential part of management (Table 13.1). Careful monitoring of growth is mandatory. The paediatrician should be a source of support, information and advice for the family. A multidisciplinary approach is needed.

 # Summary

Feeding and nutritional concerns account for a good deal of paediatric practice. You need to know what is normal in order to be able to give appropriate advice. The problems of defective nutrition are a window into our unequal world. Obesity is a problem of plenty in resource-rich countries, while malnutrition is a major

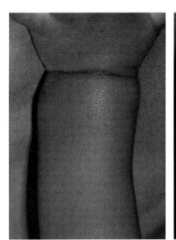
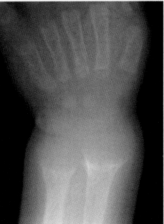
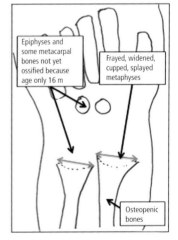

Figure 13.5 Rickets. The widened metaphyses at the distal ends of the radius and ulna can cause visible swelling of the wrist, as seen in this child.

Table 13.1 **Nutritional aspects of some childhood conditions**

Condition	Problems	Management
Severe cerebral palsy	Poor oromotor skills Gastro-oesophageal reflux Constipation Family stress Family support	Protein/energy supplements Avoid obesity Treat reflux/constipation Nasogastric/gastrostomy feeding
Cystic fibrosis	Protein fat malabsorption Recurrent infection High energy demands Loss of appetite Fat-soluble vitamins Aggressive management of infection	High energy intake (150% of average needs for age) Do not use a low-fat diet Pancreatic enzymes
Chronic renal failure	Anorexia/ill-health Renal osteodystrophy Poor vitamin D hydroxylation Poor phosphate excretion Low calcium Hyperparathyroidism	Energy supplements Nasogastric/gastrostomy feeding Controlled protein intake Phosphate restriction Vitamin D and Ca
Childhood malignancy	Anorexia Recurrent ill-health Vomiting	Protein/energy supplements Intensive nutritional support Anti-emetics

cause of childhood morbidity and mortality in poorer countries. Rickets is on the rise, and you should recognize the typical features and X-ray findings.

FOR YOUR LOG

- Ask to help make up a feed and feed some babies. Few educational activities are as delightful!
- Talk to a breastfeeding counsellor and if appropriate observe her give advice.
- Plot children's measurements (including working out and plotting BMI) on growth charts and interpret.

OSCE TIP

- Feeding problems, normal infant nutrition, weaning
- Red book and use of growth charts, e.g. failure to thrive
- Make up an infant's formula feed
- Childhood obesity: plot BMI, talk to child, talk to parent (see OSCE station 13.1).

See EMQ 13.1, EMQ 13.2 and EMQ 13.3 at the end of the book.

OSCE station 13.1: Obesity

Task: Charlie, age 8 years, has been referred because he is overweight (BMI 24 kg/m^2). His height is 75–90th centile, and his weight is over the 98th centile. His growth charts (BMI, height and weight) are provided.

  His parents are convinced that there is a 'glandular' problem. Take a history and make an initial assessment to discuss with the examiner.

Don't forget:

Is Charlie obese?	Interpret chart
Is Charlie's growth satisfactory?	Interpret height and weight together
Family history?	Do other members of the family have a similar problem?
Is diet satisfactory?	Take a brief history, a dietician will be needed to do this properly
Are there symptoms of ill-health?	Look for short stature, as well as secondary problems (e.g. poor exer-
How does obesity affect Charlie?	cise tolerance, obstructive sleep apnoea)
What does Charlie think about it?	Look for social, psychological consequences. Does he have friends, a socially supportive network? Are there problems at school?
	This is essential. Charlie needs to understand and be keen to be thinner

Charlie is obese with BMI >98th centile; he has primary obesity. His weight is above the 98th centile and his height is normal on the 75–90th centile. An endocrine problem is most unlikely. Explain a limited-calorie diet, encourage exercise and give ample moral support. Do not forbid any foods, but the second slice of buttered toast must be avoided. Charlie could join a group activity. Drugs are best avoided. Try to help alleviate any emotional stresses at home or school. If he loses weight, keep following him up for support.

SBAs

Q13.1 A child with primary obesity that you are reviewing in clinic has dark velvety patches of skin around their neck and axillae. Which co-morbidity is most likely to be associated with this finding?

a. Hypercholesterolaemia
b. Hypertension
c. Non-alcoholic Fatty Liver Disease
d. Obstructive Sleep Apnoea
e. Type 2 Diabetes

Q13.2 A 2 month old weighing 5.5 kg, who is exclusively bottle-fed is vomiting secondary to overfeeding. What volume of feed would you recommend that he has?

a. 550 mL/day
b. 825 mL/day
c. 990 mL/day
d. 1100 mL/day
e. 1210 mL/day

For SBA answers, see page 367.

14

Abnormal growth and sex development

Chapter map

Concerns about growth feature commonly in paediatric outpatient clinics, and sometimes result in admission. You need to be comfortable in assessing normal growth so that you can identify the abnormal. Common problems include failure to thrive in young children and short stature in teenagers. Problems of sex development are less common, but distressing. An understanding of the range of causes informs investigation and management.

14.1 Abnormal growth

14.1.1 Failure to thrive

14.1.1.1 What is failure to thrive?

This applies to a young child who is not growing well, usually for weight gain (Figure 14.1). In practice, this means:

- Weight crossing down through two centile lines
- Weight on or below the second centile line and falling away.

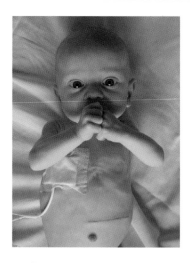

Figure 14.1 Failure to thrive. Loss of subcutaneous fat is seen in this boy who is failing to thrive.

Paediatrics Lecture Notes, Tenth Edition. Jonathan C. Darling and James Yong.
© 2022 John Wiley & Sons Ltd. Published 2022 by John Wiley & Sons Ltd.
Companion website: www.wiley.com/go/lecturenotes/paediatrics10e

Causes of failure to thrive

Inadequate food intake
- Feeding problems or neglect
- Poor appetite
- Mechanical problems, e.g. cleft palate, cerebral palsy

Vomiting
- Gastro-oesophageal reflux, pyloric stenosis
- Feeding problems
- Food intolerance

Defects of digestion or absorption
- Cystic fibrosis
- Food intolerance (including coeliac disease)
- Chronic infective diarrhoea

Failure of utilization
- Chronic infections
- Heart failure, renal failure
- Metabolic disorder

Genetically determined
- Constitutionally small
- Genetic syndrome, e.g. Turner's in girls

Emotional deprivation.

PRACTICE POINT **Common reasons for a failure to thrive referral**

- Weights measured or plotted incorrectly: do not forget to allow for gestation in the preterm (<37 weeks).
- Over the first few months of life, uterine influences 'wear off' and the child finds his own centile for weight. This may result in tracking upwards or downwards on the centile chart, and the latter may appear as failure to thrive.
- Child drinking excessive amounts of fluid – especially milk or juice. Remedy – reduce fluid intake, especially before meals.
- Poor intake and socioeconomic deprivation.

14.1.1.2 Approach to failure to thrive

Careful history and examination are essential. Sometimes the main reason for failure to thrive is obvious – inadequate food intake or chronic vomiting or diarrhoea. Often there is no clear reason apparent at the first consultation: parents appear caring and competent, adequate food is given, and there are no clues to a particular disorder. Solving the problem is difficult, and unfocused investigation is

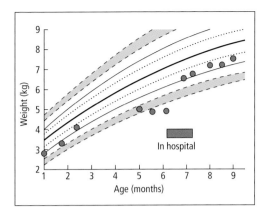

Figure 14.2 Sadie was admitted at 6 months of age with failure to thrive. In hospital, she gained weight well with normal feeding and was discharged with intensive community-based support.

not helpful. The parent-held child health record (the red book) gives invaluable information about growth. It is helpful to work with a dietician who will quantify intake and help with the management. The health visitor can provide a reliable account of the home and whether both food and emotional nourishment are available there. A home visit can be most revealing. Sometimes the child is admitted to hospital to be fed standard amounts of food and observed to see if weight gain occurs and to note symptoms (Figure 14.2). Investigations may be performed, looking for common problems first (see box). The single greatest challenge is to distinguish those with organic pathology from the many children with *non-organic failure to thrive* – an important group whose problems are social, emotional or economic in origin.

PRACTICE POINT **Investigations to consider in failure to thrive**

Depending on the severity and clinical pointers, the following may be helpful:

- Urinalysis (dipstick and microscopy and culture) – for infection
- Full blood count
- Renal and liver function
- Acute phase response (erythrocyte sedimentation rate (ESR), C-reactive protein (CRP) or plasma viscosity)
- Thyroid function
- Coeliac disease antibodies
- Chromosomes (in girls) – for Turner's.

Causes of short stature

Physiological causes
- Constitutional
- Delayed puberty

Pathological causes
- Defects of nutrition, digestion or absorption
- Social and emotional deprivation
- Most malformation syndromes
- Chronic disease (e.g. renal insufficiency, malignancy)
- Genetic syndromes (e.g. Turner syndrome in girls)
- Endocrine (e.g. deficiency of thyroid or growth hormone)
- Iatrogenic (e.g. long-term steroid therapy)
- Disorders of bone growth (e.g. skeletal dysplasias).

14.1.2   Short stature

There are many causes of short stature (see box), but the majority of children presenting with short stature are normal, short children. Some of them were born small for gestational age and many have short relatives, including one or both parents.

PRACTICE POINT   How to calculate the mid-parental height (MPH) and target centile range (TCR)

Example: Abigail has short stature, and height is on the 0.4th centile at age 11. Parents' heights: mother 154 cm, father 170 cm.

Prompts to assist you with the calculations feature on most growth charts. Essentially you are averaging the parents' heights, but adjusting for difference between the sexes.
- Reduce the father's height by mean difference between male and female heights of 14 cm. Father (adjusted) = 156 cm (170-14).
- MPH = mean of mother and father (adjusted) = 155 cm.
- TCR = MPH ± 8.5 cm.
- Plot TCR + MPH on growth chart at 18 years.
- The TCR extends to below the 0.4th centile, and her height is growing along the 0.4th centile, indicating a normal growth velocity within the target centile range.
- She is likely to be *constitutionally small*.

For boys, do the same but adjust the mother's height by adding 14 cm and calculate a slightly wider TCR by using ± 10 cm.

In healthy short children, the growth velocity is normal, as shown by serial measurements plotted on a centile chart. Growth velocity (Section 3.2.3) can be measured more accurately over 6–12 months and plotted on a growth velocity chart. The most common reason for a child being short is having short parents. The child's height centile should be compared with their 'target centile range' which is calculated from their parents' heights (see box).

Delayed puberty (often familial) with delayed bone age, i.e. their skeleton is less mature (Section 3.2.5), is common; the later pubertal growth spurt allows these children to catch up. Children whose height is below their TCR, who are obese or who have a reduced height velocity require careful assessment. Congenital hypothyroidism is detected by neonatal screening (Section 28.3.1), but acquired hypothyroidism in older children commonly presents with short stature. Growth hormone (GH) deficiency may be isolated or part of a wider pituitary insufficiency, and it may be complete or partial. Random GH levels are of little use. Diagnosis of GH deficiency requires complex tests, and secretion can only be tested by measurement after stimulation of secretion. However, it is unlikely if height velocity is normal. Bone age is delayed in both pituitary and thyroid deficiency.

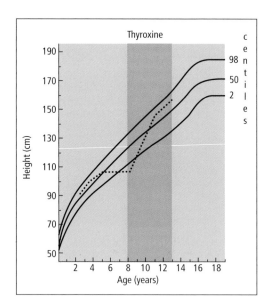

Figure 14.3 Catch-up growth. This boy developed hypothyroidism which was diagnosed at the age of 8. He showed excellent catch-up growth with replacement therapy.

Catch-up growth is seen in young children in whom the cause of retarded growth has been removed or corrected (Figure 14.3). In infants and young children, catch-up growth can be complete: thus, a 4-year-old whose growth has been suppressed by high doses of prednisolone will regain normal height once the steroid therapy is decreased or stopped. However, as puberty nears catch-up, growth may be incomplete so that temporary factors may result in permanent reduction of stature.

 PRACTICE POINT   Investigations in short stature

- Bone age (X-ray of the left wrist) (see Section 3.2.5 under Section 3.2.4)
- Thyroid function tests
- Cortisol studies
- GH stimulation test (e.g. glucagon/clonidine).

14.1.3   Tall stature

Children who are entering puberty early or who are overweight tend to be relatively tall (90–97th centile). Children with heights well above the 97th centile usually come from tall families. If height is going to exceed socially acceptable limits, exceptionally hormone therapy is used to finish the growth process prematurely.

Two important but rare causes of tall stature

Klinefelter syndrome
(see below, this chapter)
Marfan syndrome
- An autosomal dominant disorder of connective tissue.
- Features: tall and slim, arachnodactyly (long, slender fingers), typical facial appearance, prolapsing mitral valve, propensity to dislocated lenses and dissecting aneurysm of the aorta.
- When this is suspected, children should be referred for cardiology and clinical genetic review.

14.2   Abnormal sex development

14.2.1   Ambiguous genitalia

The external genitalia at birth are not clearly male or female: some are masculinized genetic females;

others are incompletely masculinized genetic males. The diagnostic problem is urgent, partly because the most common underlying disorder is dangerous congenital adrenal hyperplasia (Section 28.4.1) and partly because prolonged uncertainty about the true sex is intolerable for the parents. No-one should assign sex at birth if they are not sure; much harm may be done if the wrong sex is assigned: later reversal may be traumatic. The 'right' sex is determined by anatomy (functional possibilities), genetics and multidisciplinary discussion with the family. In some disorders of sex development, there may be ovarian and testicular tissue with indeterminate genitalia. Investigation begins with karyotyping, ultrasonography and steroid chemistry.

14.2.2   Androgen insensitivity (testicular feminisation) syndrome

The embryonic 'default' for genitalia is female unless a testosterone signal is received to switch them to male pattern during embryogenesis. Thus, abnormalities at the androgen receptor result in genetic males with testicles, but external genitalia of a female pattern. Inguinal hernias are typical, and sometimes testes are palpable in the labia majora. At puberty, normal female secondary sexual characteristics develop with amenorrhoea. Orchidectomy is advised later because of a risk of malignant change. The androgen receptor is on the X chromosome, and there is a recurrence risk for siblings.

14.2.3   Turner syndrome

Turner syndrome occurs in 1 in 2500 girls (Figure 14.4). The characteristic karyotype is 45XO (one X chromosome is lacking), but deletions or mosaicism involving the X chromosome may also be found. At birth, the only noticeable abnormality may be lymphoedema of the legs. More characteristic features may be apparent later. Coarctation of the aorta should be excluded. Secondary sexual characteristics rarely appear: the uterus and vagina may be small and the gonads rudimentary streaks in the edge of the broad ligament. Breast development and menstrual periods may be induced by hormone therapy. Affected individuals remain infertile and short (few exceed 1.5 m or 5 feet), but in some girls GH may improve stature. Intelligence is normal in most.

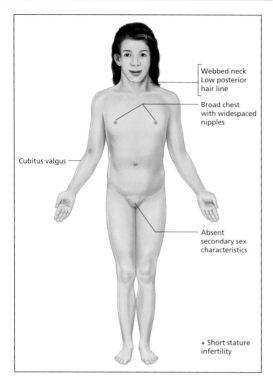

Figure 14.4 Turner syndrome.

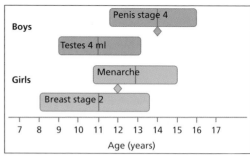

Figure 14.5 Age of puberty in boys and girls. Each bar represents the second (left-hand end) to 98th centiles, with the median shown by the vertical line in the middle of the bar. The diamonds indicate maximal growth velocity. Note that puberty starts earlier in girls, and there is an earlier growth spurt. The first sign of puberty in boys is enlargement of the testes to 4 mls, while in girls it is usually breast stage 2.

14.2.4   Klinefelter syndrome

Characteristic karyotype is 47XXY, but mosaicism may be found. Although this condition occurs in 1 in 500 males, most are not detected until late childhood or adult life. The small testicles, long limbs and female habitus are rarely noticed early in life. Spermatogenesis is always impaired, and infertility is usual.

14.2.5   Late and early puberty

Girls reach puberty on average a year before boys (Figure 14.5).

The age of puberty is influenced by genetic and environmental factors (Section 3.4).

Children (especially boys) and their parents frequently seek advice about 'late puberty'. Puberty is considered delayed if there are no signs of puberty by 13 years in a girl or 14 years in a boy. The measurement of height is useful, because physiological delay is more probable in short boys. In short girls with delayed puberty, it is important to exclude Turner syndrome. The vast majority of children with 'late' puberty are normal: they need reassurance, moral support and patience. Exceptionally, induction of puberty is indicated if there is pituitary or gonadal insufficiency.

14.2.5.1   Precocious puberty

Precocious puberty is the development of secondary sexual characteristics before 8 years in a girl or 9 years in a boy. True precocious puberty is more common in girls, while in boys it is more likely to be due to underlying pathology (e.g. brain tumour).

True (central) precocious puberty results from premature secretion of gonadotropins and follows the normal pattern of development. In gonadotropin-independent precocious puberty (e.g. congenital adrenal hyperplasia, adrenal tumours, gonadal tumours), the sequence of pubertal changes may be abnormal. Isolated precocious development of breasts (*thelarche*) is less rare and commonly resolves, followed later by normal puberty. Intracranial tumours, hydrocephalus, meningitis and encephalitis may lead to precocious puberty.

Gynaecomastia in adolescent boys is almost always physiological and self-limiting. This does not prevent it being a considerable social embarrassment.

15

Immunization and infections

Chapter map

Immunity is first lost (waning maternal antibodies) and then gradually regained, through exposure to infection and immunization. Immunization is a key public health measure of great importance to child health worldwide. Anaphylaxis is considered here because it is a rare risk when giving vaccines. Infections are a common reason for children to present to the hospital or primary care. Most are non-specific viral, but you should be able to recognize the key infective syndromes which are outlined in this chapter.

15.1 Immunity

Immunological mechanisms in childhood are essentially the same as in adults but are not fully developed at birth. Cellular immunity is effective from birth. For the first 2 or 3 years of life, the total white cell count is relatively high, and lymphocytes predominate over polymorphs in the circulating blood. Pus can be formed at any age.

Humoral (antibody-mediated) immunity is slower to develop. Maternal IgG is transferred across the placenta from early foetal life. This gives the full-term infant passive immunity to many infections, including measles, rubella and mumps. This gradually wanes from a few months to a year of age. In contrast, the larger molecules of IgM do not cross the placenta and the neonate is therefore fully susceptible to some bacterial infections including pertussis.

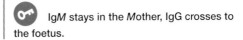 IgM stays in the *Mother*, IgG crosses to the foetus.

The foetus is capable of mounting its own IgM in response to intrauterine infection, e.g. rubella, but synthesis of other immunoglobulins gets off to a rather sluggish start after birth. Total immunoglobulin

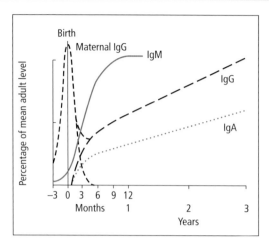

Figure 15.1 Immunoglobulin levels in early life.

 Increased susceptibility to infection

- Preterm infants
- Socio-economic deprivation
- Chronic/debilitating illness, e.g. cystic fibrosis, chronic renal failure
- Immunodeficiency, primary or secondary, e.g. treatment of malignancy
- Congenital abnormality, e.g. urinary tract anomalies.

levels in all infants are at their lowest at about 3–4 months of age, which is another susceptible period. A reasonable level of humoral immunity is established by the age of 6–9 months (Figure 15.1).

15.2 Immunization

As infectious diseases account for a large part of the mortality and morbidity of early childhood, it is essential to make the maximum use of all available preventative measures.

 PRACTICE POINT

Never miss a chance to check on, and encourage, immunization. It is every child's right to be protected against infectious diseases.

Immunization protects the individual but also prevents disease in the community. *Herd immunity* occurs with widespread immunization in the community. If a large proportion of the population is immune, the disease cannot find a host or spread. This reduces the chances of transmission of infection between children, protects any small proportion who have not had effective immunization and may even allow disease eradication (e.g. smallpox). No child should be denied immunization without serious thought as to the consequences, both for the individual child and for the community.

 Immunization – A global success story:

- a record of 123 million children immunized in 2017
- coverage for DTP sustained at around 85% of all infants
- 2–3 million deaths prevented each year
- polio nearly eradicated (only three remaining endemic countries)
- measles declined by 85% from 2000 to 2016
- neonatal and maternal tetanus eliminated in all but 14 countries by 2018

But

- 19.7 million children did not receive three doses of DTP in 2017 (Figure 15.2)
- a similar number did not receive any measles vaccine
- 1.5 million children still die each year of vaccine-preventable disease.

 RESOURCES

- https://data.unicef.org/topic/child-health/immunization/
- https://www.who.int/en/news-room/fact-sheets/detail/immunization-coverage
- For excellent visualizations on immunization coverage, see **https://data.unicef.org/resources/immunization-coverage-estimates-data-visualization/**

In Figure 15.2, the country colour indicates percentage of children vaccinated with three doses of DTP (DTP3) – see the key. The circle sizes indicate number of unvaccinated children. The largest circles are for India (2.9 m) and Nigeria (4 m) which together

Table 15.2 The vaccines

Vaccine	Protection	Nature	Live	Route
BCG (bacille Calmette–Guérin)	Tuberculosis	Attenuated mycobacterium	Yes	Intradermal
DTP	Diphtheria, tetanus, pertussis	Toxoid and bacterial antigen	No	Intramuscular or deep subcutaneous
Hep B	Hepatitis B	Recombinant	No	Intramuscular or deep subcutaneous
Hib	Haemophilus influenzae B	Conjugated capsular antigen	No	Intramuscular or deep subcutaneous
HPV	Human Papilloma Virus	Conjugated antigen	No	Intramuscular or deep subcutaneous
Influenza	Seasonal influenza	Live attenuated	Yes	Intranasal spray
Men B	Meningococcus group B	Recombinant	No	Intramuscular or deep subcutaneous
Men C	Meningococcus group C	Conjugated antigen	No	Intramuscular or deep subcutaneous
MMR	Measles, mumps, rubella	Attenuated viruses	Yes	Intramuscular or deep subcutaneous
Pneumococcus	Strep. pneumoniae	Conjugated capsular antigen	No	Intramuscular or deep subcutaneous
Polio	Poliomyelitis	Killed virus	No	Injection (has replaced oral live attenuated vaccine)
Rotavirus	Rotavirus gastroenteritis	Attenuated virus	Yes	Oral

BCG is injected *intradermally* over the insertion of the deltoid muscle. After 3–6 weeks, there is local erythema, induration and sometimes ulceration. The axillary glands may be large and painful. The local signs disappear in 2–6 months. In school children, BCG is given routinely only if the prior tuberculin skin test was negative.

15.3 Infections

Assessment and management of infection is a key skill in acute paediatrics. The presentations of infections are protean, and there are a wide range of specific and supportive therapies. Infection is by far the most common cause of acute illness.

15.3.1 Recurrent infections

Most illness in childhood is infective. In the early years of life, children meet and establish immunity to a wide variety of infecting organisms. Recurrent infections in early childhood are troublesome for children and worrying for parents, but in the vast majority of cases, the child is essentially healthy, and reassurance is all that is needed. A few children need investigation for an underlying cause such as immunodeficiency. Most recurrent infections are of the upper respiratory tract.

PRACTICE POINT Recurrent infections: when to consider further investigation

- **Failure to thrive**
- **Unusual infection**
  - More severe
  - More frequent
  - More protracted
  - Two or more episodes of pneumonia or meningitis
  - Unusual organisms
  - Unusual sites of infection.
- **Unusual features in the history**
  - Family history of immunodeficiency
  - Risk factors for HIV
  - Persistent diarrhoea.
- **Unusual features on examination**
  - Large or hard cervical or inguinal nodes, any axillary nodes
  - Hepatosplenomegaly
  - Persisting rashes.

15.3.2 Diagnosis of infections

Always begin with history, examination and then investigations. Symptom patterns and indicative signs are found in some infections. Often the presentation is non-specific. In children with unexplained fever and in some in whom a firm 'disease diagnosis' has been made (e.g. meningitis), it is important to try to establish the responsible organism.

Infection is found by:
Clinical history and findings
Identification of the organism
- Microscopy
- Culture
- PCR (polymerase chain reaction)
- Rise in specific antibody titre.

Other supportive laboratory results (e.g. CRP, white cell count).

Swabs should be taken thoroughly (especially throat swabs) and transported to the laboratory swiftly. Material for virological culture must be put straight into transport medium. Immunofluorescent techniques allow rapid, positive viral identification, e.g. rotavirus in stool, respiratory syncytial virus (RSV) in nasal secretions. Skin scrapings are needed to identify skin fungi. Demonstration of a significant rise in antibody titre, whether bacterial (e.g. anti-streptolysin O titre, ASOT) or viral, requires at least two specimens, one taken early in the illness, another 10 days to 3 weeks later. A single convalescent sample showing a high antibody titre must be interpreted more cautiously.

 Take all necessary bacteriological specimens before giving antibiotics, unless this will delay treatment that is urgently needed.

Proof of some infections (e.g. HIV, hepatitis B, meningococcus and pertussis) may be possible by polymerase chain reaction (PCR) tests which detect the relevant DNA/RNA material and provide a rapid result.

15.3.3 Infections in childhood

15.3.3.1 Important childhood infectious diseases

Table 15.3 shows key characteristics of important childhood infectious diseases. In general, infectivity

antiretroviral treatment, but the decline is slowing, and also for new infection rate in adolescents. Infection from blood products still occurs in developing countries. Infected babies appear normal at birth, but without prophylaxis nearly 25% develop AIDS or die in the first year. The rest show a much slower disease progression, with some showing no evidence of indicator diseases (e.g. pneumocystis carinii pneumonia) until the teenage years.

Conditions that suggest AIDS

- Opportunist infection
- Recurrent bacterial infections
- Failure to thrive
- Encephalopathy
- Malignancy.

The HIV antibody test is unreliable in infancy because of maternal antibody transmission. Children over 18 months who have HIV antibody are infected. PCR tests for viral RNA are increasingly used for diagnosis. Prophylactic treatment is begun as soon as HIV infection is suspected, and some units give prophylaxis to all children born to HIV-positive mothers from birth.

HIV: reduction of vertical transmission

- Maternal antiretroviral therapy in pregnancy
- Caesarean section
- Avoid breastfeeding (in developed countries)
- Antiretroviral treatment for infant in first weeks
- UK vertical transmission rate of 0.3% in 2014 (in 2/3rds of these UK cases, diagnosis of HIV in the mother is made after delivery)

15.3.3.3 Bacterial infections

Meningococcal disease

The Gram-negative diplococcus (*Neisseria meningitidis*) (meningococcus) is divided into several serogroups: groups B and C are most prevalent in the UK (Figure 15.6).

Meningococcal disease is most often seen in infants and young children, although there is a second peak in 15–19 year olds. Despite the significant impact of meningococcal immunization (see above), it remains an important cause of morbidity in the UK (nearly 800 cases per year) and has a case fatality rate of just over 10%. Transmission is via close contact with nasopharyngeal droplets. Infections are more common in winter. The peak incidence is at 6–8 months of age, with a smaller second peak in teenagers (of whom 25% are nasopharyngeal carriers). The incubation period is 2–10 days. The presentation varies according to the dominance of either septicaemia or meningitis.

Meningococcal infection

- 25% septicaemia
- 60% septicaemia and meningitis
- 15% meningitis alone.

Septicaemia

 PRACTICE POINT

A young child may be well in the morning and dead in the evening as a result of meningococcal septicaemia.

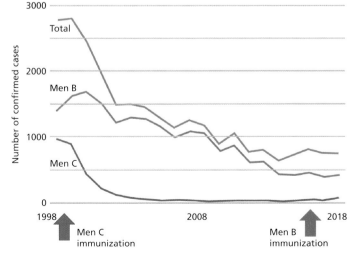

Figure 15.6 Meningococcal disease: annual confirmed cases in England and Wales. Source: Based on Public Health England and the UK Health Protection Agency Archive.

Mild non-specific symptoms are followed within days, or within hours (in severe cases), by severe illness and fever and the rapid appearance of a widespread red, macular rash which soon becomes purpuric (not blanching on pressure) (Figure 15.7). The rash may be sparse or profuse. Typically, it appears before your eyes. It varies from tiny petechial spots to large purpuric lesions which coalesce to form large ecchymoses. Septic shock follows in 30% of cases and requires prompt diagnosis and treatment. Severely ill children require treatment in a paediatric intensive care unit; others can be treated safely with antibiotics and antipyretics on the children's ward.

(a)

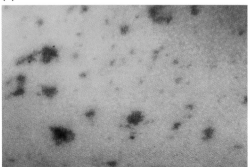

(b)

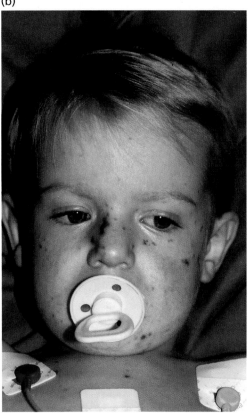

Figure 15.7 (a and b) Meningococcal rash. Make sure you can recognize this rash. Recognition saves lives.

 PRACTICE POINT

A feverish ill child who has a purpuric rash should immediately be given benzylpenicillin IV or IM and then transferred urgently to hospital.

Meningococcus may be grown from pharyngeal swab, blood culture, aspirate of skin lesions or CSF. PCR tests provide confirmation of diagnosis.

There is an increased risk of disease in the child's close contacts at home or in the nursery, though such secondary cases are rare. Close contacts are given a single dose of Ciprofloxacin (as is the affected child before leaving hospital) to lessen the risk of such secondary infection.

Meningococcus is the most common cause of bacterial meningitis in Europe (features are described in Section 18.5.1).

Tuberculosis

Tuberculosis is common wherever poverty, malnutrition and overcrowding are prevalent, and rare where standards of hygiene and nutrition are good. It is the leading cause of death from a single infectious agent worldwide (above HIV), with one-fifth of deaths occurring in HIV positive people. Ten percent of all new cases are in children. The chief sources of infection are adults with sputum-positive pulmonary tuberculosis (*Mycobacterium tuberculosis*) and milk from infected cattle (*Mycobacterium bovis*). Erythema nodosum may be caused by tuberculosis (Section 25.2.8).

In Europe, childhood tuberculosis is becoming more common again. Primary complexes in the lung are seen more often in immigrant children from Asia than in others.

The WHO estimates an annual incidence of over 10 million cases of TB in the world, of whom 95% live in developing countries. The WHO 'End TB strategy' aims to reduce TB deaths by 90% between 2015 and 2030. Early detection of infection and treatment is key.

Prevention depends first upon general improvement in socio-economic conditions, and secondly upon specific measures including the prompt recognition and treatment of infectious adults, BCG immunization, tuberculin testing of cattle and pasteurization of milk.

> 1.6 million of the world's population die from TB each year.

The initial infection is in the lungs if conveyed by droplets, or in the bowel if conveyed by milk. The first site of infection is known as the *primary focus*. The *primary complex* comprises the primary focus and the enlarged lymph nodes draining it. Spread of infection beyond the local nodes may result in tubercle bacilli reaching the bloodstream, causing either tuberculous septicaemia (*miliary TB*- Figure 15.8) or infection of distant organs (meninges, kidneys, bones and joints). Tuberculous cervical lymph nodes are thought to be infected via the tonsils.

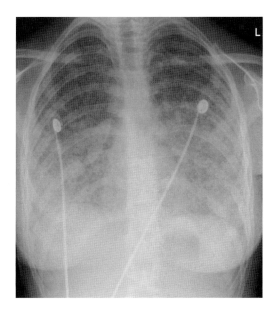

Figure 15.8 Miliary TB. This 13-year-old Asian girl presented with several weeks of cough, fever, shortness of breath and weight loss, and was later confirmed to have TB. Her X-ray shows florid reticulo-nodular infiltrates throughout the lung fields consistent with miliary TB (the term 'miliary' was originally used because the multiple small lesions resemble millet seeds).

The child with a primary complex has minimal symptoms. Haemoptysis and systemic symptoms are exceptional. Children with TB, traced through their contact with infected adults, are often symptom-free. Diagnosis is based on X-ray appearances and a positive tuberculin test. Sputum is not usually present, but tubercle bacilli may be recovered from gastric washings.

Tuberculous meningitis

This disease is dangerous and may lead to death or permanent disability. The onset is insidious and diagnosis difficult, with weight loss, vague malaise, anorexia and perhaps slight fever. Evidence of meningeal involvement may be shown by headache, drowsiness, irritability and neck stiffness. Later, there may be convulsions, focal neurological signs and impairment of consciousness.

 PRACTICE POINT

A child with lymphocytic meningitis, and low CSF glucose, should be treated for TB until proved otherwise.

Cervical adenopathy

Tuberculous neck glands are rare in the UK. Unilateral, firm lymph nodes are characteristic. In TB, the tuberculin test is positive.

 PRACTICE POINT **Diagnosis of TB**

Tuberculin test
- Intradermal tuberculin is injected in the forearm.
- A skin reaction occurs if child has been exposed to TB.
- Size of reaction checked 2–3 days later.
- Children who have been immunized should have some reaction.
- Strong reaction indicates active TB.

Chest X-ray may show lesions of pulmonary TB
PCR, e.g. on CSF sample
Bacterial culture – slow (several weeks)
Gastric washings may yield the organism.
TB blood tests based on the immune response to the bacteria (interferon-gamma release) are increasingly useful.

Management

Regardless of the site, the management of tuberculosis can be divided into three parts.

Notification of the case: immunization of contacts and identification of possible sources.

Anti-tuberculous drugs: rifampicin, pyrazinamide and isoniazid form the basis of treatment. Treatment should be continued for at least 6 months. Drug-resistant TB is reaching crisis levels in some countries.

General management: children should not be admitted to the hospital or kept off school without good reason. A pulmonary primary complex is rarely infectious, and isolation is unnecessary. If nutrition is unsatisfactory, it should be improved.

15.3.3.4 Other infections/infection-like syndromes

Malaria

Malaria and international child health

About half the world's population is at risk of malaria (Figure 15.9), with the major mortality burden concentrated in Africa, and in children under 5. Malaria accounts for one in five of all childhood deaths in Africa. It is a major cause of childhood anaemia, which leads to poor growth and development. Maternal disease leads to low birthweight infants. The WHO leads a global campaign to eliminate malaria, with special focus on around 20 countries close to eliminating the disease. The focus is on proven strategies: insecticide-treated nets, rapid diagnostic tests, prompt treatment of malarial disease and treatment of pregnant women.

Malaria is endemic in many parts of the world and may be seen in immigrants from malarious areas or in persons who have visited such places within the preceding 4 months. It usually presents with fever, which does not necessarily show the classic periodic pattern. The spleen may be enlarged. The gold standard for diagnosis is microscopy of thick and thin blood films to identify parasites. However, rapid diagnostic tests based on antigen detection are increasingly available and don't require laboratory facilities and expertise.

 PRACTICE POINT

Think of malaria in the ill febrile child with a positive travel history.

There is increasing concern about *Plasmodium* drug resistance. Artemisinin-based combination therapy is usually the recommended treatment, but this may vary according to the local sensitivity of the responsible organism. Prophylactic drugs must be taken throughout residence in a malarial area and for at least 4 weeks afterwards (Figure 15.9).

Kawasaki disease

This is a rare but important disease. It presents as a systemic febrile vasculitis affecting children under the age of 5. No causative organism has been identified. It is the most common cause of acquired heart disease in childhood in developed countries (where rheumatic fever is rare). Coronary arteritis leads to the formation of aneurysms in up to 30% of children, which can be fatal.

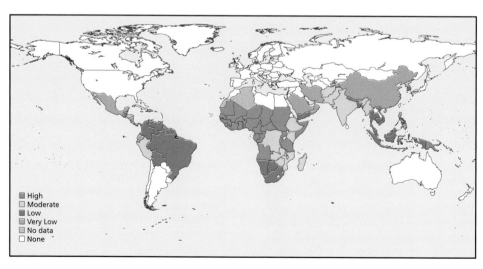

High
Moderate
Low
Very Low
No data
None

Figure 15.9 Distribution of malarial endemic areas by CDC estimated risk. *Source:* Figure from Treated.com (used with permission). Data sourced from CDC, July 2018: https://www.cdc.gov/malaria/travelers/country_table/a.html

SBAs

Q15.1 Amy's parents bring her to the GP to discuss MMR immunization. She is age 13 months, and they have followed the normal immunization course so far, but they have come across social media sites which link MMR to autism. She also has egg allergy. She currently has a runny nose but no fever. They are not sure whether she should have the MMR immunization.

What is the most appropriate evidence-based advice?

a. Egg allergy is a contraindication to MMR, and she should not have the immunization.

b. She has an upper respiratory infection, so the vaccine should be deferred. Please return in two weeks.

c. There is evidence that MMR causes autism, and the immunization should be avoided.

d. There is no evidence of a link between MMR and autism. Egg allergy is not a contraindication. Any small risks of immunization are far outweighed by the benefits. She should have the immunization.

e. There is no evidence of a link between MMR and autism. She should have had the MMR immunization with her earlier course of immunizations at 2–4 months, but it is not too late and she should have it now.

Q15.2 You see a 15-month-old boy Edward in a paediatric clinic. His parents are very worried about his recurrent upper respiratory infections – he has about 1 a month. He has two school-age siblings and attends a nursery. His growth since birth has been along the ninth centile for weight, length and head circumference. He is otherwise well. On examination, he has about four smooth mobile cervical lymph nodes, two on each side, measuring 0.5 cm each. His parents have not noticed these before. Otherwise, examination is normal.

What is the most appropriate management?

a. Advise his parents to stop sending him to nursery

b. Advise his parents you are concerned about his growth only being on the ninth centile

c. Arrange an USS of his neck

d. CXR and full blood count

e. Reassure his parents that he is normal.

Q15.3 Nazir age 2 years has had a fever of 38 degrees C on and off for 5 days and has been irritable with red eyes (no pus) and a rash on his trunk (now resolved). On examination, he has very red, cracked lips, several cervical nodes measuring 1.5–2.0 cm bilaterally, and mildly swollen fingers.

What is the most appropriate treatment?

a. Intravenous immunoglobulin and oral aspirin

b. Intravenous penicillin

c. Oral paracetamol

d. Oral penicillin

e. Reassure and encourage oral fluids

For SBA answers, see page 367.

16

Accidents and non-accidents

Chapter map

Accidents are common and important. Non-accidents are rarer and are part of the spectrum of child abuse. This chapter will describe the main types of both. Although sudden infant death syndrome does not fit either category, there are areas of overlap.

16.1 Accidents

Accidents are a common cause of death in children over the age of 1 year (Section 1.3.2). The number of child deaths due to accident in the UK has been declining steadily for 40 years from over 1000 to around 130 currently; 70% are boys. Every year over two million children are taken to a hospital after having an accident.

Accidents vary by age group:

- Road traffic accidents involve mainly children of school age (about 60 deaths per year in the UK, 3% of all road deaths).

- Accidents in the home involve mainly children under the age of five (also about 60 deaths per year in the UK).

 Most common causes of home accidents

- non-fatal - falls
- fatal - fire.

The risk of accident is influenced by social circumstances. The child in a large family in poor housing, on the street much of the day and ostensibly supervised by another child only marginally older, is at great hazard; and the lone-parent trying to care for young children at the top of a tower block, without the privilege of an enclosed garden or play space, has a difficult task.

> Children of parents who have never worked, or who have been unemployed for a long time, are 13 times more likely to die from unintentional injury than children of parents in higher professional occupations.

Pedestrian accidents are most common in the 5–9 age group when parents are falsely confident about their child's skills: it is wiser to underestimate, rather than overestimate a child's abilities. In general, children cannot cross a busy road safely, even at a traffic light, on their own until the age of 8 or 9 years, and cannot ride a bicycle safely on a main road until 13.

There is a great need for better education of children and parents about safety, and for legislation to minimize the opportunities for accidents (Figure 16.1).

> The UK government has targeted accident prevention as a key policy area over the past 40 years, and there has been a steady reduction in number of accidents in children. However, accidents remain one of the leading causes of morbidity and mortality in childhood.

 Button batteries

Keep small batteries away from children – when swallowed they can erode tissue (e.g. to puncture the aorta)

 RESOURCE

Child Accident Prevention Trust (**https://www.capt.org.uk**) provides prevention-focused resources for parents and professionals
Royal Society for the Prevention of Accidents (**https://www.rospa.com**) is more general and aims to prevent all accidents

16.1.1 Head injury

 KEY POINTS

- Apparently, trivial injuries can lead to intracranial bleeding that only becomes clinically apparent after an interval of time
- Intracranial bleeding may occur without a skull fracture
- CT head scan is the first-line investigation after significant head injury.

16.1.1.1 Management

- Airways, Breathing and Circulation
- Observe
  - pulse

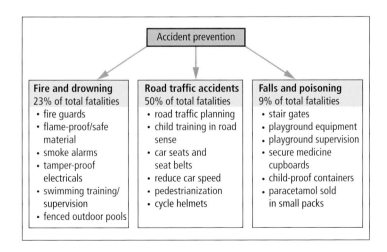

Figure 16.1 Accident prevention.

Accident prevention		
Fire and drowning 23% of total fatalities • fire guards • flame-proof/safe material • smoke alarms • tamper-proof electricals • swimming training/ supervision • fenced outdoor pools	**Road traffic accidents** 50% of total fatalities • road traffic planning • child training in road sense • car seats and seat belts • reduce car speed • pedestrianization • cycle helmets	**Falls and poisoning** 9% of total fatalities • stair gates • playground equipment • playground supervision • secure medicine cupboards • child-proof containers • paracetamol sold in small packs

- respiratory rate
- blood pressure
- level of consciousness
- pupillary size and reactions
- CT head scan if risk factors for serious intracranial injury (Figure 16.2)
- Consider spinal imaging (X rays +/− CT depending on suspicion and severity of injury)
- Admit and observe (usually overnight) if:
  - severe injury
  - any neurological symptom or sign including depressed conscious level
  - persisting symptoms:
    - headache
    - vomiting
    - altered behaviour
- Consider non-accidental injury if injuries and history don't match, or other suggestive features (Section 16.2).

RESOURCE

National guidelines for the management of head injury in children and adults (CG 176) are available at **www.nice.org.uk**. These or similar are used by most A&E departments.

16.1.2   Burns and scalds

16.1.2.1   Scalds

- Caused by hot fluids
- Predominantly loss of epidermis
- Blistering
- Peeling.

The skin of young children sometimes suffers full-thickness loss from comparatively minor scalds. There is a strong argument for limiting the maximum temperature of hot water in the home to 54 °C (129 °F). Most scalds occur in the kitchen.

16.1.2.2   Burns

- Caused by
  - direct contact with very hot objects
  - clothes catching fire
- Often full-thickness skin loss
- Shock – fluid is lost through the damaged skin surface (Figure 16.3).

If more than 10% of the body surface is involved, intravenous fluid therapy will be required. Burns involving 50% or more of the body surface carry a grave prognosis, although children have survived more extensive burns than this.

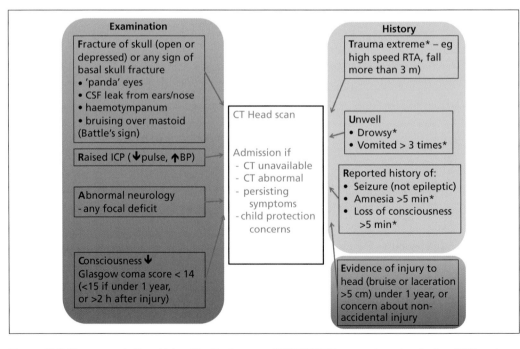

Figure 16.2 Management of head injury. Use the Acronym 'FRACTURE' to remember when to do a CT Scan in a child with head injury if any feature present (for asterisked features, more than one needs to be present). *Source:* Based on Head injury: assessment and early management, NICE guideline CG98, 2014.

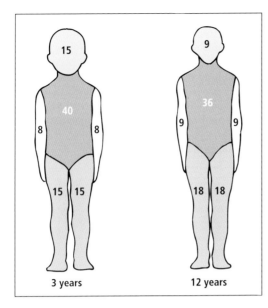

3 years | 12 years

Figure 16.3 Skin surface areas at 3 and 12 years. The figures indicate the percentage of total body surface represented by each part.

 PRACTICE POINT

Burns and scalds are more serious than they seem, and hospital admission is advisable for all but the most trivial. Severe injury needs specialized multidisciplinary care in a Burns unit.

16.1.2.3   Prevention

- Use cordless kettles or with short coiled flexes (reduces risk of child reaching up and pulling the kettle over)
- Place pans on back of hob, handles turned inwards
- Take care of children in the kitchen or use door gate to keep children away when cooking
- Run cold water into bath before hot water
- Fireguards, radiator guards
- Smoke alarms.

16.1.3   Poisoning

16.1.3.1   Accidental poisoning

- Common
- Many substances (Table 16.1)

Table 16.1 Substances children swallow accidentally

Tablets and medicines	Household and horticultural fluids	Berries and seeds
Sleeping tablets	Bleach	Laburnum
Tranquillizers	Turpentine	Deadly nightshade
Antidepressants	Paraffin	Toadstools
Iron	Cleaning fluids	
Analgesics	Weedkillers	

- Toddlers aged 2–4 years
  - agile enough to find and swallow things
  - do not appreciate the dangers
- Less than 15% of children develop symptoms
- Death is very rare.

In the UK, things plucked from the hedgerows and ditches hardly ever cause serious illness.

16.1.3.2   Deliberate poisoning

Older children may ingest drugs to self-harm, or recreationally (see Section 17.4.1), while rarely children may be deliberately poisoned by parents or carers (Table 16.2).

16.1.3.3   Management

 PRACTICE POINT

- Identify poison
- Check with poisons information centre
- Estimate maximum amount/toxicity
- Minimize absorption (activated charcoal absorbs the poison – but used not for alcohols, metal salts, corrosives)
- Specific antidote
  - Paracetamol – acetylcysteine
  - Iron – desferrioxamine chelates iron, thus reducing absorption
  - Opioid – naloxone reverses (may need to be repeated)
- Specific techniques to enhance elimination (rarely)
  - Haemodialysis
  - Alkalinise urine for salicylates
- Combat symptoms
- Admit poisoned children to the hospital for observation for at least a few hours

Table 16.2 Characteristic patterns in different types of poisoning

	Accidental	Self-harm	Deliberate (by parent)
Occurrence	Very common	Common	Uncommon
Age (years)	2–4	>10	0–5
Substance	Anything	Analgesic	Prescribed drug
Quantity	Small	Variable	Large
Recurrence risk	Small	Medium	Large

 TREATMENT   Paracetamol poisoning

- May cause liver necrosis (maximal at 3–4 days) and renal damage
- May be few symptoms at first
- Transfer to hospital urgently if >75mg/kg ingested
- Activated charcoal
- Measure level after 4 h and plot on treatment graph
- Acetylcysteine iv protects the liver and is given if
  - level above treatment line
  - presentation 8–24 h after ingestion
  - some staggered overdoses
- Liver function tests, creatinine and INR guide further treatment

 RESOURCE

Toxbase (**www.toxbase.org**) – an online resource for the NHS – should be consulted for any poisoning.
  The National Poisons Information Service **www.npis.org** is available for more detailed expert help and advice. (Contact details are in the British National Formulary and the BNF for Children.)
  The BNF for Children **https://bnfc.nice.org.uk** has a useful section (search 'Poisoning').

16.2   Child abuse and neglect

 Abuse: deliberately inflicted injury.

Neglect: inadequate or negligent parenting, failing to protect the child.

Many children suffer a combination of abuse and neglect. The definitions suggest that abuse is an active process and neglect a passive one, but for most forms of abuse, the parents, who are the usual perpetrators, contribute to the abuse by both active and passive roles (Figure 16.4). Thus, the spouse who fails to intervene when their partner sexually abuses the child is a passive partner to the abuse and colluding with it. A parent who passively fails to provide food or love may also indulge in active physical assault.

Types of abuse
- Physical abuse
- Neglect
- Sexual abuse
- Emotional abuse
- Factitious and induced illness (Munchausen syndrome by proxy).

A child is considered to be abused if he or she is treated by an adult in a way that is unacceptable in a given culture at a given time. It is important to recognize that children are treated differently not only in different countries but in different subcultures of one city and that there will be various opinions about what constitutes abuse. With the passage of time, standards change: corporal punishment is much less acceptable than it was. These factors contribute to the difficulties of determining changes in the prevalence of abuse.

16.2.1   Physical abuse (non-accidental injury)

This is usually short-term and violent, though it may be repetitive. Infants and toddlers are most at risk. Soft tissue injuries to the skin, ears and eyes are common, as well as injuries to the joints and bones (Figure 16.5).

16.2.1.1   Common patterns of injury

- Bruising
  - especially face and trunk
  - multiple
  - different ages

Note: a normal active toddler will often have five or six bruises of different ages, usually on the shins

- Fractures
  - especially ribs, humerus and femur (Figure 16.6)
  - different stages of healing denote repetitive injury
  - infants do not often sustain accidental fractures
  - often no clear history

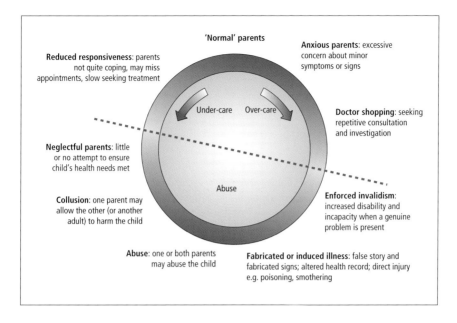

Figure 16.4 The spectrum of parental behaviour towards illness.

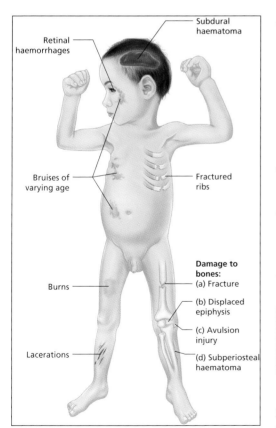

Figure 16.5 Characteristic injuries caused by physical abuse.

- Head injuries
  - due to direct injury or shaking (shaken baby syndrome)
  - skull fracture
  - subdural haematoma
  - fractures especially if depressed or complicated (as opposed to simple linear)
  - retinal haemorrhages
  - severe, intracranial haemorrhage leads to death or permanent brain damage
- Burns
  - cigarettes
  - holding a child close to a fire
- Scalds
  - immersion in very hot water
  - usually involve hand, foot or buttock.

16.2.2   Neglect

> **Neglect**
> - Failure to provide the love, care, food or physical circumstances that will allow the child to grow and develop normally
> - Exposing a child to any kind of danger.

Neglect and injury are closely associated, and both are indications of parental inadequacy. The child may show evidence of poor standards of hygiene or nutrition; height and weight, when plotted on a growth

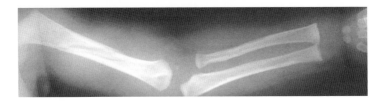

Figure 16.6 Spiral fracture of the humerus in a young child. These are often caused non-accidentally due to wrenching and twisting forces across the limb, and there may be little or no history of any significant injury.

record, may be well below the expected centile (*non-organic failure to thrive*: 14.1.1.2). Neglect is often combined with emotional abuse.

 Features suggesting non-accidental injury

- Delay in seeking medical advice
- Explanation incompatible with injury (a baby's skull does not fracture if he rolls off the sofa onto a carpeted floor)
- Story varies
- Child brought by someone other than the person in whose presence the injury occurred
- Unusual parent or child behaviour
- Parents more interested in their own feelings, and in returning home, than in concern for the child
- Abnormal parent–child interaction, with the child looking frightened or withdrawn.

16.2.3   Sexual abuse

Child sexual abuse includes any use of children for the sexual gratification of adults. It ranges from inappropriate fondling and masturbation to intercourse and buggery. Children may be forced to appear in pornographic photographs or videos, or participate in sex rings or ritual abuse. *Organized abuse* is the term used to describe abuse involving either a number of children, or a number of abusers. In *child sexual exploitation*, the child or young person is given gifts, drugs, status or affection in return for sex – often preceded by a phase of grooming. It can happen in person or online.

16.2.3.1   Presentations of sexual abuse

- Disclosure by child or carer
- Local
  - trauma
  - infection
  - perineal soreness
  - discharge or bleeding

- sexually transmitted infections
- pregnancy
- Behaviour change
  - anorexia
  - encopresis/enuresis
  - self-harm
  - sexual behaviour inappropriate for the child's age or environment
  - alcohol/drug abuse
  - secretive
  - having unexplained money or gifts.

Children of all ages, and either sex, are abused, though the most common is for a girl to be abused by a male who is either a relative or a member of the household.

 Female genital mutilation

This involves pricking, cutting or other harm to the genitalia of a young girl, and is practised in some parts of Africa, the Middle East and Asia. It is illegal in the UK, with mandatory reporting – if it is identified by a health professional, they must report it.

16.2.4   Emotional abuse (psychological abuse)

> The child receives the repeated message that he is worthless, unloved or unwanted, or only of use in meeting the parents' needs.

Emotional abuse ranges from the failure of parents to provide consistent love, to overt hostility including spurning, terrorizing, isolating, corrupting and exploiting, or merely denying the child the right to emotional responsiveness. For an infant, this may result in failure to thrive with recurrent minor infections and frequent attendances at hospitals and health centres, general developmental delay and a lack of social responsiveness. The older child is likely to be short, developmentally immature and with delayed language skills. Her behaviour is likely to be overactive, impulsive and aggressive. All abuse entails some emotional ill-treatment, but currently, it is uncommon for emotional abuse alone to be the sole reason for child protection measures through legal action, even though its consequences can be more severe than occasional episodes of physical abuse.

16.2.5 Factitious or induced illness

This term encompasses a range of behaviour in which false illness in the child is invented or induced for the benefit of the abuser. It commonly includes both physical and emotional abuse. The harmful behaviour lies at the far end of the spectrum of inappropriate ways in which parents may behave in relation to childhood illness. It may present as a 'perplexing presentation'.

The consequences for the child can be disastrous:

- Unpleasant and harmful investigations and treatments
- Induction of genuine disease
- Effects of poisoning or suffocation
- Longer-term effects on child
- Child assumes illness role, believes himself to be disabled
- Misses school
- Somatoform or factitious behaviour (e.g. Munchausen syndrome) as an adult.

16.2.6 Prevalence of child abuse and neglect

- One in five children have experienced severe maltreatment
- Physical abuse affects about 8%; neglect 15%; emotional abuse 7%; and sexual abuse up to 25% (5–10% penetrative abuse in girls)
- One in three children sexually abused didn't tell anyone at the time

There is some evidence that there may have been an increase in child abuse in recent years, but the apparent increase may be more the result of greater unwillingness by society to tolerate child abuse, increased public awareness and professional recognition.

16.2.7 Perpetrators

- Most child abuse occurs in the home
- The parents are the usual abusers
- Physical abuse, emotional abuse and neglect are often inflicted by both parents

- Sexual abuse is more common by fathers/step-fathers
- Poisoning, smothering and factitious and induced illness are most commonly perpetrated by the mother.

Abuse occurs in all sections of society, but probably occurs more commonly in poor families. Abused deprived children are more likely to become abusing, neglecting parents – *the cycle of deprivation.*

The motives for abuse are complex. We can all understand how a weary parent in an overcrowded home, where the children are on top of one another, and the father is on shift work attempting to sleep, hits out impatiently at a fractious overdemanding child. However, much abuse is repetitive and, seemingly, premeditated. Often it is an expression of the parent's inner violence and their wish to exert power over their child. It is common for normal parents to have mixed feelings about their children and to have moments when they hate their child. Most parents can control their feelings, but a minority injure their child during those feelings of hatred. Most are not suffering from mental illness.

16.2.8 Management of child abuse and neglect

Unless you think of the possibility of abuse, you won't diagnose it. When you suspect abuse, you need to know what action to take, and where to refer for more detailed assessment. Know about local policies and referral routes (usually general or community paediatric departments, and/or social services).

 TREATMENT

In suspected abuse, consider the following:
- Record history carefully (and who provided it) – always!
- Sketch of injuries
- Photographs
- Skeletal survey (X-rays of skull, chest and limbs)
- CT head scan
- Ophthalmology review for retinal haemorrhages
- Blood clotting screen if bruising.
- Check whether known to social services
- Seek advice from local safeguarding professionals.

Multidisciplinary involvement is key to all steps in management. The following may be asked to provide information, or be involved in the discussion:

- Child
- GP

- Parents
- Health visitor
- School nurse
- Family
- Hospital staff
- Neighbours
- Social services
- School/nursery
- Police.

If abuse is likely, the doctor (or another concerned person) will contact the Social Services Department who usually convene a case conference (Figure 16.7). The aim is to form a clear picture of the child and family relationships. Then, making the child's interests paramount, recommendations are made for the child's future safety, including decisions about future legal proceedings.

If the child is in imminent danger, police protection powers may be used, or an *Emergency Protection Order* may be sought from a magistrate. This allows the child to be detained in a hospital or foster home whilst enquiries are made. In view of the high incidence of abuse in siblings, it is mandatory to check the other children in the child's home. Subsequent court action may be needed to take a child into the care of the local authority if the risk of further abuse at home is too great (Section 1.6).

More commonly the child is made subject to a *Child Protection Plan* and skilled help arranged for the families so that the child can be supervised at home and the family helped to modify their behaviour. This help and supervision are normally provided by local authority social workers or the *National Society for the Prevention of Cruelty to Children (NSPCC)*. Further abuse occurs in up to 20% of cases; the recurrence rate is a sensitive index of the effectiveness of management.

The police are represented at case conferences and may be asked to investigate more serious or difficult cases. Only a minority of cases end with a criminal prosecution.

 PRACTICE POINT Difficult conversations about safeguarding

There is no easy way to talk about safeguarding concerns with parents, for example when there is an unexplained serious injury in a young child who needs to be admitted for further investigation and assessment. In general, a firm, clear but sympathetic approach is followed, which may include the following points:
- There is an injury that raises concerns about intentional harm to the child
- In these situations, we are required to follow a safeguarding process
- The child is kept at the centre
- Investigations such as X-rays may be needed (these are explained)
- The child may need to stay in the hospital while tests are done
- Decisions are made jointly with other agencies, particularly social services and police

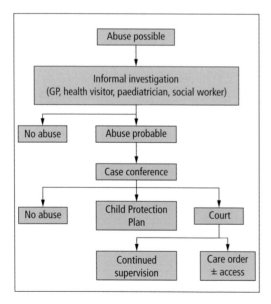

Figure 16.7 The usual course of investigation of alleged child abuse.

 RESOURCE

The NSPCC (**https://learning.nspcc.org.uk**) provides a useful range of resources.

'Working together to safeguard children' is the statutory UK guidance document on safeguarding. Go to **www.gov.uk** and search for 'Working together'.

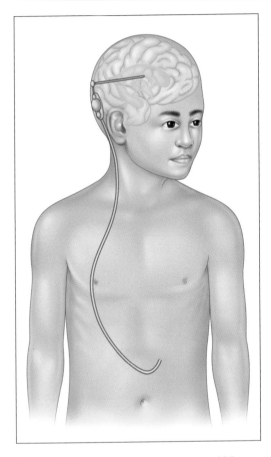

Figure 18.7 If hydrocephalus is progressive, CSF can be drained from the lateral ventricle to the peritoneal cavity. The ventriculo–peritoneal shunt is tunnelled under the skin and can be felt behind the ear.

Spina bifida is due to failure of closure of the posterior neuropore, which normally occurs around the 27th day of embryonic life.

The most common and most severe form is a *meningomyelocele* (myelocele) in which elements of the spinal cord and nerve roots are involved. It may occur at any spinal level, but the usual site is the lumbar region. The baby is born with a raw swelling over the spine in which the malformed spinal cord is exposed.

It is often associated with hydrocephalus, particularly as a result of the *Arnold–Chiari malformation* where the cerebellar tonsils protrude into the foramen magnum, blocking flow of CSF from the fourth ventricle.

The emotional and social problems for the child and family are considerable, varying from the

 Meningomyelocele

- Legs – paralysis with sensory loss below the level of the lesion, hip dislocation and leg deformities (club foot).
- Head – hydrocephalus with learning problems.
- Bladder – neuropathic bladder with incontinence, recurrent urinary tract infections and renal damage.
- Anus – faecal incontinence.

frequent hospital admissions and attendances to the problems of providing suitable education for a paraplegic, incontinent child. Children with this condition need the care of a large multidisciplinary team. Foetal detection usually leads to termination of pregnancy.

18.7.2   Meningocele

This is rare and less serious. The swelling over the lower back is covered by skin and contains no neural tissue. Cosmetic surgery is not urgent.

18.7.3   Encephalocele

Encephaloceles are protrusions of brain through the skull, covered by skin, usually in the occipital region. They are often associated with severe brain abnormality.

18.7.4   Spina bifida occulta

Minor defects of the posterior arches of the lower lumbar vertebrae are common and do not matter at all. Sacral dimples in the natal cleft are normal. Intraspinal pathology is rare but slightly more likely if there are external 'markers' in the lumbar region (hairy tuft, naevus, lipoma). The main concern is tethering of the spinal cord, which may result in traction on the cord as the child grows.

18.8   Cerebral palsy

A disorder of posture and movement resulting from a non-progressive lesion of the developing brain.

Incidence is two in 1000. The basic pathology may be a developmental abnormality, pre- or postnatal brain infection, physical or chemical injury to the brain, or a vascular accident (Figure 18.8). The brain lesion is fixed and non-progressive, but the clinical picture changes with CNS maturation. A hypotonic neonate may become hypertonic during the first year of life.

Presentation varies according to severity. In the severe cases, poor sucking or altered muscle tone is present soon after birth. More often cerebral palsy is suspected during the first 2 years. Follow-up surveillance of high-risk newborns (e.g. extreme preterm delivery, birth asphyxia) aims to allow earlier detection and intervention.

> **Causes of cerebral palsy**
>
> **Prenatal**
> 70% primary brain malformation; congenital viral infection (Section 9.4.4)
>
> **Perinatal**
> 15% birth asphyxia; trauma; stroke
>
> **Postnatal**
> 15% intraventricular haemorrhage and periventricular leukomalacia (preterm); meningitis; trauma; metabolic.

> **PRACTICE POINT**
>
> CP presents with the following:
> • Delayed motor development
> • Gait problems
> • Feeding difficulties
> • Hand preference in infancy
> • Abnormal movements.
> These presentations also have many other potential causes.

Figure 18.8 This brain MRI shows a neonatal stroke which led to a hemiplegic cerebral palsy.

18.8.1 Classification (Figure 18.9)

Cerebral palsy covers a very broad spectrum of disability, ranging from problems playing football to complete dependency. Classification across axes

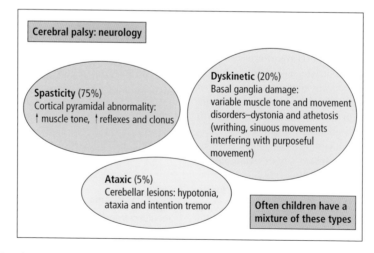

Figure 18.9 Neurology of cerebral palsy.

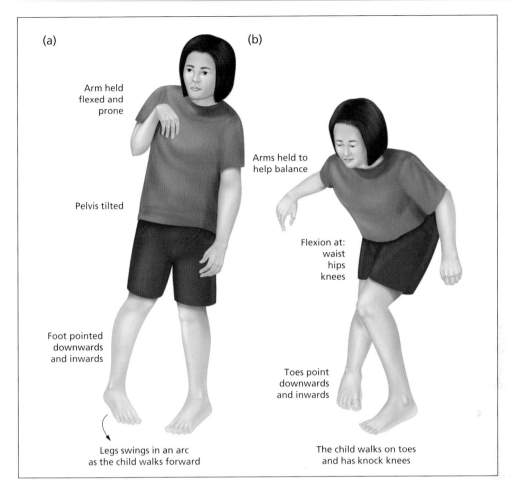

(a)

Arm held flexed and prone

Pelvis tilted

Foot pointed downwards and inwards

Legs swings in an arc as the child walks forward

(b)

Arms held to help balance

Flexion at:
waist
hips
knees

Toes point downwards and inwards

The child walks on toes and has knock knees

Figure 18.10 Abnormal gaits in children with (a) hemiplegia and (b) diplegia.

> **Terminology in cerebral palsy**
>
> *Diplegia*. Predominant involvement of the legs, though the arms may also be affected.
> *Quadriplegia*. Involvement of all four limbs.
> *Hemiplegia*. Involvement of one arm and one leg on the same side (Figure 18.10).

(including pattern, severity, disability, associated problems and cause) assist care and support of the individual child.

18.8.2 Management

Early comprehensive assessment and where necessary investigation is essential because of the following:

- Other disability is common in learning difficulties, epilepsy, defects of vision and hearing and behavioural problems.
- Disordered posture and movement can lead to permanent deformities.
- Cerebral palsy can present major problems at home and at school.

Assessment, family support and therapy are organized by the multidisciplinary team in the *Child Development Centre*. Early physiotherapy (and sometimes botulinum toxin injections) aims to establish a normal pattern of movement and to prevent deformity. Orthopaedic surgery may correct deformity to improve function. Speech therapy is needed for feeding and speech. The team also includes occupational therapist (aids, wheelchairs), educational psychologist and health visitor/social worker. Usually, the community paediatrician takes a leading role.

18.8.3 Prognosis

This depends mainly on the pattern and severity of CP, associated handicaps, and in particular on the intelligence of the child. With normal intelligence, the problems of even severe motor handicaps may be overcome. The quality of the management itself affects the prognosis. A severely affected child may require education in a special school where expert physiotherapy, occupational therapy, teaching and other facilities are available.

Children less severely affected, often those with hemiplegia, manage at normal school. The least severely affected of all do not always reach the specialist. Their clumsiness or educational problems may not be recognized as mild cerebral palsy.

18.9 Headaches

 If headache wakes the child at night, is present on waking or worse in the early morning, this may mean raised intracranial pressure. Brain imaging may be needed.

Headaches are a common outpatient symptom but are unusual in younger children.

> PRACTICE POINT **Causes of headaches**
>
> - Stress/tension
> - Migraine
> - Eye strain
> - Dental problems
> - Sinusitis
> - Space-occupying lesion

18.9.1 Stress headaches

- Common
- Daytime
- Not present on waking

- Timing relates to stress (school, etc.)
- Frontal
- No associated symptoms.

18.9.2 Migraine

Migraine is classically unilateral, the headaches are throbbing in nature and associated with nausea or vomiting and photophobia; a visual aura is much less common in children than in adults with migraine. Migraine sometimes results from sensitivity to food (chocolate, cheese) or food additives. It is unusual to diagnose migraine in the absence of a family history.

18.10 Space-occupying lesions

Symptoms vary greatly in pattern, severity and timing. Headache, misery and irritability are common early symptoms and are followed by unsteadiness, vomiting and visual disturbances. Fits may occur.

> **Space-occupying lesions**
>
> - **Neoplasm**
> - **Subdural haematoma**
>   - Accidents
>   - Non-accidental injury, shaking (Section 16.2.1)
> - **Cerebral abscess**
>   - Meningitis
>   - Infected emboli (Section 21.5.4.1)
>   - Chronic otitis media.

> PRACTICE POINT
>
> If a space-occupying lesion is suspected, CT or MR brain imaging must be carried out promptly (Section 27.3).

Focal seizures or signs should always make you think of a space-occupying lesion. Management demands a multidisciplinary approach including paediatrics, neurology, radiology and neurosurgery.

18.11 Abnormal head shape

18.11.1 Craniosynostosis (craniostenosis)

Premature fusion of one or more of the skull sutures results in an unusual-shaped head and may compress the brain or cranial nerves. The prognosis depends upon which sutures are affected. Premature fusion of all sutures results in a bulging forehead, proptosis and brain compression, and requires surgery. Syntostosis of a single suture may require surgery for cosmetic reasons. The cause is unknown. Sometimes, there is a hereditary factor with associated skeletal abnormalities.

18.11.2 Plagiocephaly and skull flattening

Natural skull asymmetry is common in early infancy, but the sutures and fontanelles are normal. In the more obvious plagiocephaly, one side of the forehead and occiput are displaced forward (Figure 18.11). The asym-

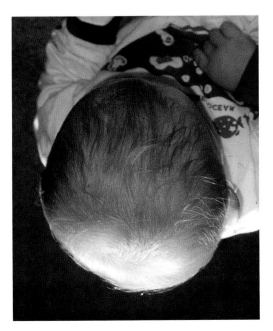

Figure 18.11 Plagiocephaly. The left forehead is more prominent than the right, while the left occiput is flattened.

metry becomes less with growth and does not cause problems. There may be associated chest asymmetry.

Flattened occiput is common in infants nursed on their backs and resolves with time. Head shaping helmets preserve shape but have no medical benefit.

18.12 Progressive neuromuscular disorders

Among the most distressing disorders of childhood are those that strike a previously healthy child and progress inexorably towards incapacity and death over months or, more often, years. They may affect principally the brain, the spinal cord or the muscles; many are genetically determined and few are open to effective treatment. Onset is usually in the first 2 years; in general, the earlier the onset, the more rapid the progress.

> 🔑 The clinical hallmark is loss of previously acquired skills.

Progressive brain degeneration conditions are often due to autosomal recessive genes (Section 6.2.1). They can be grouped into those that affect the grey matter (e.g. the *lipidoses* such as *Tay–Sachs disease*) and those that affect the white matter (*leucodystrophies*).

18.12.1 Spinal muscular atrophies

- Autosomal recessive
- Proximal muscle weakness
- Tongue fasciculation
- Normal facial movement
- Variable age of onset and progression.

The infantile form (*Werdnig–Hoffmann disease*) is evident from birth and progresses to death within a year or so; forms with later onset progress more slowly. Those with a condition with onset in late childhood enjoy a reasonably active adult life.

18.12.2 Myopathies (muscular dystrophies)

The muscular dystrophies vary in their age of onset, rate of progress and mode of inheritance.

18.12.2.1   Duchenne muscular dystrophy

This is the most common type of muscular dystrophy. It only affects boys because it is due to an X-linked recessive gene. The genetic abnormality is a deletion in the gene for dystrophin, a protein essential for muscle function. The condition presents at 1–6 years with difficulty walking, an abnormal waddling gait or difficulty climbing stairs. Affected boys develop enlargement of the calves due to fatty infiltration (*pseudohypertrophy*) with absent knee jerks. There is often marked lumbar lordosis.

The ability to walk is lost at about the age of 10 years, and death occurs in early adulthood due to pneumonia or myocardial involvement. A proportion have intellectual impairment. A grossly elevated serum creatine phosphokinase level is present, and genetic testing is diagnostic.

> In Duchenne dystrophy, boys asked to stand up from sitting on the floor turn over onto all fours, and then 'climb up their legs'. This is Gower's sign (Figure 3.11).

There is no cure for the dystrophies, and therapy is supportive as follows: physiotherapy, prevent deformity and maintain mobility. Obesity is to be avoided. Clinical and genetic diagnosis allows genetic counselling and antenatal diagnosis in future pregnancies. Research focuses on gene therapy or modulation.

In a milder form of pseudohypertrophic muscular dystrophy (*Becker*), symptoms develop later and disability is mild.

18.12.3   Other progressive disorders

18.12.3.1   Rett syndrome

- Severe mental and physical handicap in girls
- Normal early development
- Slow psychomotor development by 1 year
- Loss of manipulative skills and speech
- Repetitive hand movements, e.g. hand wringing.

Many progressive neuromuscular diseases of adult life have their onset in childhood. Examples are *myotonic dystrophy* (which may be lethal in the newborn) and *Friedreich's ataxia*.

18.13   The floppy infant

Degrees of infantile hypotonia are common and usually resolve with maturation. Infants present with poor head control, floppiness or feeding problems. In severe hypotonia, there is paucity of movement and respiratory problems.

> When picked up under the arms the baby tends to slip from one's grasp. In ventral suspension, the baby flops like a rag doll.

Floppy infants fall into two main groups.

18.13.1   Benign hypotonia

Temporary floppiness characterized by gradual improvement over months. There may be a helpful family history.

18.13.2   Paralytic with weakness

Severe weakness accompanies hypotonia in conditions due to spinal or muscular disease. These infants make few movements and may be unable to raise their arm upwards against gravity. It can be caused by a number of rare neuromuscular or spinal cord disorders (e.g. spinal muscular atrophy, see above).

18.13.3   Non-paralytic without weakness

Hypotonia with mild weakness. Possible causes include the following:

- Severe/neurodevelopmental delay
- Cerebral palsy – children with spasticity are initially floppy
- Certain syndromes – Down, Prader–Willi (obesity, hypotonia, hypogonadism)
- Systemic disorders – malnutrition, rickets and hypothyroidism.

Summary

Neurological problems in a developing foetus, infant or child may have lifelong consequences. You should know about fits, cerebral palsy and meningitis, and understand a little about the wide spectrum of neurological disorders. All are very worrying for the child and her family: while many resolve, a few are progressive and even lethal. For more severe conditions, the key is early detection, accurate diagnosis, and access for the child and family to the multidisciplinary team.

 FOR YOUR LOG

- Febrile fits are a common cause for admission to see when you are on call.
- Talk to a child or family who have had fits or have epilepsy.
- Visit the Child Development Centre or community based neurodisability team.
- Attend a multidisciplinary meeting.
- Ask to visit a child with cerebral palsy at home during your GP attachment.

 OSCE TIP

- 'Tommy was admitted with a febrile fit last night. He now appears well. Please talk to his mother about febrile fits'.
- Function, tone, power and reflexes in the lower limbs (see OSCE station 17.1).
- Manikin: management of the fitting child.
- Video: recognize epileptic seizures and non-epileptic events.
- Results of a lumbar puncture.
- Cerebral palsy: assess gait, type of cerebral palsy, limb distribution.
- Examine gait, coordination, cognitive function.

See EMQ 18.1, EMQ 18.2, EMQ 18.3, and EMQ 18.4 at the end of the book.

OSCE station 18.1: Neurological examination of the legs

Clinical approach:

- Observer for other neurological or neurodevelopmental problems
- Is the child generally alert and aware?
- Is she behaving as you would expect?

Gait
- Ask mother/child if happy to walk
- Best to observe in underwear, no shoes
- Observe for:
  ◊ Which part of foot strikes floor
  ◊ Right and left leg movements
  ◊ Symmetry
  ◊ Position of rest of body

Inspection
- Muscle wasting
- Muscle hypertrophy
- Asymmetry
- Limb shortening
- Scars (e.g. lumbosacral, lengthening of TAs)

Tone
- Assess tone at hips, knees, and ankles
- Don't forget hip adductors and plantarflexors
- Clonus

Power
- What does gait and movement tell you?
- Power at hip, knee and ankle

Reflexes
- Knee jerks — if absent try reinforcement
- Ankle jerks
- Plantar response

Beth has difficulty walking. She is 4 years old. Please examine her legs for tone and power walks with:
- Flexed knees and hips
- Inturned feet
- Toe stepping
- No heel strike

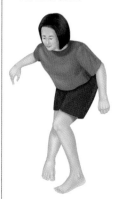

No marks or scars on back

tone ↑ in legs especially:
- Hip adductors
- → scissoring
- Plantar flexors
- → Toe pointing

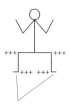

Sustained clonus

Beth has spastic cerebral palsy. When legs are affected more than arms, this is a diplegia.

Never forget:

- Say hello and introduce yourself
- General health
- Colour — ?pale/?cyanosed
- Quickly assess growth, nutrition and development
- Mention the obvious (e.g. drip, leg in plaster)

Look around for:

- Shoes — Piedro boots
- Look at soles of shoes for pattern of wear
- Ankle–foot orthoses
- Walking aids
- Evidence of urinary or faecal problems

Special points

- If the child is willing/able, begin by asking the child to walk, and then to sit on the floor and get up, then use the tendon hammer
- Use MRC classification of power if you wish but you do not need to
- Show children what you want them to do or give simple explanations

SBAs

Q18.1 A 3-year-old girl ran into a chair and hurt her leg. There was no crying, but she went quiet and pale and quickly collapsed to the floor and became very stiff. There was then some jerking which lasted for a 'few seconds', and then her colour returned and she was conscious after about 2–3 min.

What is the most appropriate management?

a. Buccal midazolam
b. Electrocardiogram (ECG)
c. Electroencephalogram (EEG)
d. MRI head
e. Sodium valproate

Q18.2 A 7-year-old boy presents with a history of worsening headaches that wake him at night, and he has some early morning vomiting. He has no focal neurology on examination but is noted to be hypertensive

What would be the most appropriate next step?

a. Advise to avoid cheese and chocolate
b. Lumbar puncture to check opening pressures
c. Simple analgesia for headaches
d. Trial with Pizotifen
e. Urgent CT/MRI head

For SBA answers, see page 367.

19

Ear, nose and throat

Chapter map

ENT problems are very common in children. The upper respiratory tract is the most common site of infection in the young child, and assessment of acute illness is not complete without examination of the ears, nose and throat (Section 3.5.2). Chronic disorders are important causes of long-term morbidity. The early diagnosis of sensorineural and conductive hearing loss is essential if educational and social effects are to be minimized (Section 11.4.5). Often more serious or chronic disorders are managed together with a paediatric ENT surgeon.

> 🔑 Children are now vaccinated against *Streptococcus pneumoniae* and *Haemophilus influenzae*: two important causes of ENT infection.

19.1 Ear problems

19.1.1 Otitis media

Acute otitis media is common throughout the first 8 years. In the older child, the cardinal symptom, earache, makes detection easy; in infants, it may not be so obvious. They usually have high fever and are irritable, rolling their heads from side to side or rubbing their ears. There is a red, bulging, painful tympanic membrane, which may lead to perforation and discharge of pus. A mildly pink dull drum may be present in any upper respiratory tract infection (URTI).

A majority of otitis media is viral, but distinction from bacterial infection is difficult. The evidence indicates that simple analgesia is all that is needed in most cases, but antibiotics (amoxicillin) should be given if the child is very unwell, vulnerable (e.g. through immunosuppression or prematurity) or if symptoms persist for more than 3 days. Paracetamol is invaluable for the fever and pain. Persistent aural discharge (chronic suppurative otitis media) is a potential complication. To prevent further episodes, ensure pneumococcal immunizations are up to date, and avoid passive smoking, dummies (pacifiers) and supine feeding.

> **Rare important complications**
> - Mastoiditis
> - Lateral sinus thrombosis
> - Meningitis
> - Cerebral abscess.

Paediatrics Lecture Notes, Tenth Edition. Jonathan C. Darling and James Yong.
© 2022 John Wiley & Sons Ltd. Published 2022 by John Wiley & Sons Ltd.
Companion website: www.wiley.com/go/lecturenotes/paediatrics10e

RESOURCE

NICE guideline NG91 **https://www.nice.org.uk/ guidance/ng91**

19.1.2 Otitis media with effusion (glue ear, secretory otitis media)

Glue ear is the most common cause of conductive hearing loss below the age of 10 years (Figures 19.1– 19.3). Sticky, serous material accumulates in the middle ear insidiously or after acute otitis media. The symptoms are deafness, speech delay, and older children may report a feeling of fullness or popping in the ear. It is especially common in children who have atopy, frequent upper respiratory infections or cleft

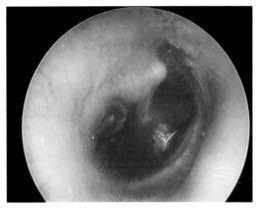

Figure 19.3 The drum is dull and retracted in otitis media with effusion. *Source:* Lindsey C. Knight.

palate. The eardrum is usually dull and retracted, and a fluid level may be seen. The malleus handle is more horizontal and appears shorter, broader and whiter. Antibiotics, antihistamines and decongestants may be tried. If there is significant deafness, an indwelling tube (*grommet*) is inserted through the eardrum to aerate the middle ear and is left for 6–12 months.

Hearing impairment is covered in Section 11.4.5.

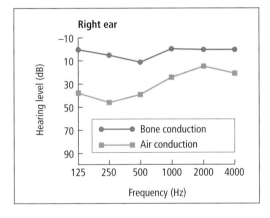

Figure 19.1 Audiogram: this child has right, moderate, conductive hearing loss.

19.2 Nose and sinuses

19.2.1 Sinusitis

The frontal and sphenoidal sinuses do not develop until 5 and 9 years, respectively. The maxillary and

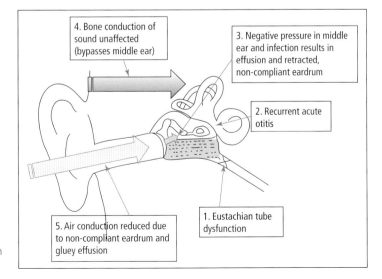

4. Bone conduction of sound unaffected (bypasses middle ear)

3. Negative pressure in middle ear and infection results in effusion and retracted, non-compliant eardrum

2. Recurrent acute otitis

1. Eustachian tube dysfunction

5. Air conduction reduced due to non-compliant eardrum and gluey effusion

Figure 19.2 Otitis media with effusion.

ethmoidal sinuses are small in these years and sinusitis is uncommon before the age of 5.

19.2.2 Allergic rhinitis

Recurrent bouts of sneezing, a persistent watery nasal discharge and watering eyes are typically worse outside in bright sunshine. The nasal mucosa is pale and oedematous. Hay fever is allergic rhinitis in late spring and early summer in response to grass pollen.

> **TREATMENT**
>
> If you are giving antihistamines, use non-sedating medication. You may need to warn teenagers about alcohol and sedation.

Other allergens include dust, animal dander and moulds. A careful history is more likely to identify the allergen than allergy tests. Nose and eye drops are useful. Therapeutic success with antihistamines and topical steroids is variable.

19.2.3 Epistaxis

Nose bleeds usually originate from the anterior inferior corner of the nasal septum (Little's area). Common causes are minor injury and URTIs. Children may alarm everyone by vomiting blood which they have swallowed. First aid consists of sitting the child up and squeezing the nose firmly, whilst the child is comforted and told to breathe through the mouth.

19.3 Throat

19.3.1 Tonsils and adenoids

Lymphoid tissue grows rapidly in the first 5 years of life. Tonsils and adenoids are usually small in infants and reach their greatest relative size between 4 and 7 years.

> **PRACTICE POINT**
>
> Examine a young child's neck carefully, and you will find palpable lymph glands. Learn what normal glands feel like (Section 3.5.1, p. 36), so you will recognize enlargement due to infection.

19.3.1.1 Acute tonsillitis

This is very common in the age group 2–8 years but uncommon in infants. There is sudden onset of fever, sore throat and dysphagia. Vomiting and abdominal pains are common. The tonsils are enlarged and fiery red; white exudate appears in the tonsillar glands.

> **Rare important complications**
>
> **Immediate**
> - *Peritonsillar abscess (quinsy)*: severe symptoms of tonsillitis and dysphagia. The tonsil is displaced towards the midline. If suspected, refer to ENT that day.
> - *Cervical abscess*: infection localizes in a cervical lymph gland
>
> **Delayed**
> - *Acute nephritis* (Section 23.4.2): 2–3 weeks later
> - *Rheumatic fever* (Section 24.3.6): 1–2 weeks later.

Tender cervical lymphadenopathy is usual. Viral and bacterial tonsillitis cannot be distinguished clinically. The most common bacterial pathogen (30–40%) is β-haemolytic streptococcus. Infectious mononucleosis is associated with nasty tonsillitis in older children.

Paracetamol, cool drinks, and local anaesthetic throat spray can provide symptomatic relief. Don't routinely prescribe antibiotics. For persistent or severe symptoms, penicillin may be used to eradicate streptococci and reduce the risk of complications.

> **Cervical lymphadenopathy: differential diagnosis**
>
> - Reactive (e.g. tonsillitis) – vastly more common than any other cause
> - TB
> - Malignancy (lymphoma, leukaemia) – glands craggy, hard, tethered
> - Other infections (e.g. glandular fever, rubella, atypical mycobacteria, toxoplasma).

Cervical glands with recurrent tonsillitis are usually bilateral, fairly soft and mobile, and only rarely form a localized abscess. In most school-age children, some cervical nodes are palpable.

19.3.1.2 Obstructive sleep apnoea

In rare cases, enlargement of the tonsils or adenoidal tissue causes upper airway obstruction. This leads to difficulty in breathing, with loud snoring and a disturbed abnormal pattern of breathing during sleep. It is more common in obesity. The result of disturbed sleep is tiredness during the day and behavioural problems. In severe cases, poor growth and development and a wide variety of symptoms are seen, and occasionally the nocturnal hypoxia may lead to pulmonary hypertension. Recognition is important: ask about snoring and consider overnight pulse oximetry. Tonsillectomy/adenoidectomy gives good results.

19.3.1.3 Adenotonsillectomy

 TREATMENT **Indications**

- Mastoiditis
- Recurrent/persistent tonsillitis (>3 attacks a year)
- Obstructive sleep apnoea
- Recurrent otitis media.

Tonsillectomy is not performed to prevent children catching colds, sore throats or bronchitis: it does not improve the child's appetite or growth. In the right children, the results are very good.

19.3.2 Stridor

In young children, the larynx is small with walls that are flabby compared with the firm, cartilaginous adult larynx. It is a voice bag, not a voice box, and it collapses and obstructs easily.

> Stridor is mainly inspiratory and is the noise due to upper airway obstruction, usually in the larynx.

19.3.2.1 Laryngomalacia

Laryngomalacia is a form of congenital stridor due to floppy aryepiglottic folds. It does not cause serious obstruction and gradually disappears as the laryngeal cartilage becomes firmer during the first year of life. If it is severe enough to cause intercostal and suprasternal recession, or feeding problems, or if there is no improvement in the first weeks, laryngoscopy is advisable.

19.3.2.2 Acute stridor

In young children, especially infants and toddlers, stridor can progress to serious respiratory obstruction with alarming rapidity. If in doubt, admit. The main causes of acute stridor are:

1 Acute laryngotracheitis (croup)
2 Foreign body in the larynx (Section 20.5.4)
3 Epiglottitis.

 PRACTICE POINT

In acute stridor with respiratory distress, do not examine the throat: you may precipitate complete airway obstruction.

19.3.2.3 Acute laryngotracheitis (croup)

Croup

- Age 1–4 years
- Mild/moderate systemic illness
- Viral infection
- Associated URTI
- Stridor and barking cough.

This is common, often mild, but sometimes alarming and potentially dangerous. Onset is sudden, often at night, with stridor, harsh cry and a barking cough (croup). Mild cases, with no stridor at rest, can be managed at home. Admit more severe cases, and those under 6 months, or distant from hospital. If obstruction is marked, there may be intercostal and suprasternal recession in addition to stridor. Monitor severe cases carefully. If you think airway obstruction may be imminent, experts who can intubate are needed. A 'croup score' can be used to rate overall severity and guide management.

 TREATMENT

- Treat with steroids: oral dexamethasone or nebulized budesonide
- Antibiotics not usually indicated
- Some need intravenous fluids
- Nebulized adrenaline provides temporary benefit in severe croup
- Intubation rarely needed.

19.3.2.4 Epiglottitis

This life-threatening disease is prevented by immunization against *Haemophilus influenzae* (Chapter 15). This child with stridor is acutely ill and feverish, with a muffled cough. In this serious emergency, the child's airway is in grave danger of complete obstruction: she sits up, drooling because swallowing is difficult. At intubation, the swollen epiglottis may be seen like a cherry. Associated septicaemia is common, and prompt antibiotic and supportive treatment are essential.

 Summary

Acute ENT infection is a common cause of presentation to primary care and hospital, so it is important to look for it in any child with a fever. Most infections are viral and do not need antibiotic treatment unless severe, persisting for several days or unusual. Beware of the child with stridor, especially if you suspect epiglottitis.

 OSCE TIP

- Examine ENT – practice correct positioning of child (see Section 3.5.2)
- Manikin: examine ears and make diagnosis of otitis media, etc.

 FOR YOUR LOG

- Examine ears and throat in young children as far as you are able without causing upset. Remember correct positioning is important, and you can always practice this. You can also practice on a manikin.
- Palpate cervical lymph nodes routinely when you examine children.

See EMQ 19.1 at the end of the book.

SBA

Q19.1 A 2-year-old boy is brought to the Emergency Department in the early hours with a 2 hour history of increasing difficulty breathing. He has been unwell for 2 days with an upper respiratory infection, and increasing cough which is barking or 'seal-like' in quality. On examination he appears well, temperature is 37.5°C, and he has inspiratory stridor when active but not at rest, with signs of mild respiratory distress. His chest is clear, and respiratory rate mildly elevated. His oxygen saturations are 97% in air.

What is the most appropriate first line treatment?
- **a.** Adrenaline (nebulized)
- **b.** Amoxicillin (oral)
- **c.** Dexamethasone (oral)
- **d.** Oxygen (by facemask)
- **e.** Salbutamol (nebulized)

Q19.2 Eleanor age 11 months attends her GP surgery with an emergency appointment. She looks unwell, has a temperature of 40°C and is drooling with a muffled cough. She has inspiratory stridor. Her parents have declined all immunizations for her. The GP is concerned and calls an ambulance.

What is the most likely organism causing her symptoms?
- **a.** Haemophilus influenza B
- **b.** Neisseria meningitidis
- **c.** Pneumococcus
- **d.** Respiratory syncytial virus
- **e.** β-haemolytic streptococcus

Q19.3 Tanvir aged 2½ years has had recurrent upper respiratory and ear infections for the past year. His parents are concerned about poor hearing and speech delay. On examination he appears well, but both tympanic membranes are dull and retracted, with no light reflexes, and fluid levels visible. Audiogram shows reduced air conduction bilaterally. This situation persists and the ENT surgeon advises insertion of bilateral grommets.

What is the most appropriate summary of the mechanism by which the grommets work?
- **a.** Amplify movements of the ossicles
- **b.** Conduct sound into the middle ear
- **c.** Drain fluid from the middle ear
- **d.** Equalize the pressure across the tympanic membrane
- **e.** Reduce pressure in the middle ear

For SBA answers, see page 368.

20

Respiratory medicine

Chapter map

Respiratory infections and asthma are major causes of morbidity and are common reasons for a child being taken to a doctor or admitted to hospital. Certain problems are more common at certain ages, and the same organism may cause different illnesses at different ages (e.g. respiratory syncytial virus (RSV) causes bronchiolitis in infants, and a cold or a sore throat in older children). Cystic fibrosis is one of the commonest life-threatening genetically inherited conditions in the Caucasian population. Early recognition and careful paediatric management greatly improve outcome, and we are on the threshold of new 'step-change' treatments.

20.1 Symptoms of respiratory tract disease

Cough in children is usually an upper respiratory tract infection (URTI) and less often lung disease. A barking cough suggests a laryngeal or tracheal disorder, usually croup (see Table 20.1). Young asthmatics may cough instead of wheeze, especially at night. Children usually swallow their sputum unless it is copious. Purulent and blood-stained sputum are rare. Earache (manifested by pulling at the ear in young children) suggests acute otitis media, although remember that pain from lower back teeth may be referred to the ear.

Paediatrics Lecture Notes, Tenth Edition. Jonathan C. Darling and James Yong.
© 2022 John Wiley & Sons Ltd. Published 2022 by John Wiley & Sons Ltd.
Companion website: www.wiley.com/go/lecturenotes/paediatrics10e

Table 20.1 Respiratory symptoms and their causes

Symptom	Causes	Character
Cough	Croup	Barking
	URTI	Throaty
	Asthma	Worse at night
	Pneumonia	Productive of phlegm (but children usually swallow this)
	Bronchiolitis	RSV cough unpleasant with characteristic 'wet' sound
	Pertussis	Paroxysms of coughing, ending with inspiratory 'whoop', persists many days
Shortness of breath	Asthma	
	Pneumonia	
	Bronchiolitis	
Noisy breathing		
Stridor (*a monophonic noise arising from the upper airway, usually inspiratory*)	Croup	Accompanied by barking cough
	Foreign body	History of inhalation or choking?
	Epiglottitis	Muffled cough, drooling, high temperature
		Rare since Hib vaccine
		If suspected, don't examine throat
Wheeze (*a polyphonic musical noise arising from the bronchi/ bronchioles, usually more expiratory than inspiratory*)	Asthma	Widespread
	Pneumonia	Focal
	Inhaled foreign body	Focal
	Bronchiolitis	Widespread, with inspiratory crackles in under-2 s
Snuffles/nasal obstruction	URTI	
Ruttles/rattles	Mucus 'rattling' in large airways	

Respiratory distress and failure

Recognition of severe respiratory disease is essential. Intervene before respiratory distress leads to respiratory failure.

Respiratory distress (increased work of breathing)

- Tachypnoea (>50/min infants; >40/min in children)
- Intercostal/subcostal recession
- Use of accessory muscles (arms and shoulders)
- Expiratory grunting, nasal flaring and 'head-bobbing' in infants

Respiratory failure (respiratory effort insufficient or unsustainable)

- Severe respiratory distress or
- Diminished respiratory effort, apnoea
- CNS signs of hypoxia: agitation; fatigue; drowsiness
- Cyanosis
- Collapse.

20.2 Upper respiratory tract

Most illnesses of childhood are infections; most childhood infections are respiratory; and most are URTI (Table 20.2). The incidence and type of respiratory infections vary with age (Figure 20.1).

PRACTICE POINT

Don't forget to examine the ears, nose and throat in febrile children – unless you suspect epiglottitis (see Section 19.3.2.4)!

In the infant, nasal obstruction due to the common cold may lead to feeding difficulties. Saline drops and gentle suction can remove obstructing mucus plugs from the nostrils, but decongestant drops should be

Table 20.2 **Upper respiratory tract infection (URTI)**		
Infection	**Description**	**Causes**
	All may cause fever, vomiting and anorexia	*The great majority are viral*
Common cold	Cough, rhinitis, sneeze	Viral
Tonsillitis	Enlarged, inflamed tonsils, +/– exudate	Viral or bacterial
Pharyngitis	Inflamed throat	Viral or bacterial
Acute otitis media	Earache, inflamed and bulging tympanic membrane	Viral or bacterial

Persistent cough

Common
- Postinfective
- Run of recurrent URTIs
- Postnasal drip
- Asthma (exercise, night)
- Cigarette smoke
- Habit

Uncommon
- Pertussis
- Foreign body
- Gastro-oesophageal reflux
- Cystic fibrosis
- Tuberculosis
- Immune deficiency.

avoided. Eustachian tube obstruction often causes earache, and the eardrums may appear congested. Antibiotics are not indicated. Paracetamol will reduce fever and relieve discomfort.

URTI may precipitate febrile convulsions (Section 18.1.1) and asthma attacks and is sometimes the precursor of acute specific fevers, especially measles (Table 15.3) or bronchiolitis.

20.2.1 Recurrent coughs and colds

Recurrent coughs and colds, sometimes with sore throat and earache, are very common in young children, particularly if they have older school-age siblings, or mix with other children in a nursery. Some babies and toddlers are catarrhal much of the time. The first winter at school or nursery is frequently punctuated by upper respiratory infections.

Poor social circumstances and passive smoking predispose to catarrh. Some children will not blow their noses; some with severe nasal obstruction cannot. Aromatic inhalations and rubs can be useful in older children, but should be avoided in young infants, particularly under 3 months. Decongestants and cough suppressants are not recommended. The best healer is the passage of time.

20.3 Apnoea

Temporary cessation of breathing is a frightening occurrence. It can result from central respiratory depression or from mechanical obstruction (including the inhalation of food or vomit). It may occur during the first day or two of respiratory infections, particularly pertussis or RSV. However, many infants

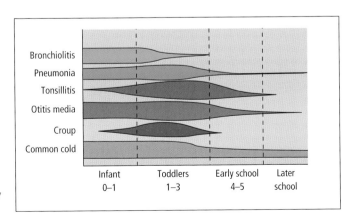

Figure 20.1 Incidence of respiratory infections.

Table 20.3 Clues to alternative diagnoses in wheezy children

Clinical clue	Possible diagnosis
Perinatal and family history	
Symptoms present from birth or perinatal lung problem	Cystic fibrosis; chronic lung disease of prematurity; ciliary dyskinesia; developmental lung anomaly
Family history of unusual chest disease	Cystic fibrosis; neuromuscular disorder
Severe upper respiratory tract disease	Defect of host defence; ciliary dyskinesia
Symptoms and signs	
Persistent moist cough	Cystic fibrosis; bronchiectasis; protracted bacterial bronchitis; recurrent aspiration; host defence disorder; ciliary dyskinesia
Excessive vomiting	Gastro-oesophageal reflux (with or without aspiration)
Paroxysmal coughing bouts leading to vomiting	Pertussis
Dysphagia	Swallowing problems (with or without aspiration)
Breathlessness with light headedness and peripheral tingling	Dysfunctional breathing, panic attacks
Inspiratory stridor	Tracheal or laryngeal disorder
Abnormal voice or cry	Laryngeal problem
Focal signs in chest	Developmental anomaly; postinfective syndrome; bronchiectasis; tuberculosis
Finger clubbing	Cystic fibrosis; bronchiectasis
Failure to thrive	Cystic fibrosis; host defence disorder; gastro-oesophageal reflux
Investigations	
Focal or persistent radiological changes	Developmental lung anomaly; cystic fibrosis; post-infective disorder; recurrent aspiration; inhaled foreign body; bronchiectasis; tuberculosis

Source: From the Scottish Intercollegiate Guidelines Network (SIGN) guideline 'British guideline on the management of asthma'. Edinburgh: SIGN; 2019. (SIGN publication no. 158). Available from URL: http://www.sign.ac.uk Used with permission.

are rushed to the hospital by their parents, who believe their child has stopped breathing. Often it is not clear whether anxious parents have merely misinterpreted the normal variable breathing of a small baby, or whether the baby genuinely has had a significant spell of apnoea. When the apnoea is associated with cyanosis, or unconsciousness, the differential diagnosis must include a seizure, congenital heart disease or airways obstruction. For parents who have suffered a previous sudden infant death, the loan of an apnoea alarm, which sounds when the baby stops breathing, may be comforting. However, evidence that it prevents a future occurrence is lacking. Most children who die suddenly and unexpectedly in early life have not had previous spells of apnoea.

20.4   Influenza

Influenza tends to occur in epidemics, affecting particularly school children and young adults. The general symptoms of high fever, headache and malaise tend to overshadow the dry cough and sore throat, though there may be signs of pharyngitis, tracheitis or bronchitis. The main complications result from secondary bacterial infection of lungs, middle ear or sinuses. The brief incubation period and high infectivity favour massive outbreaks. Immunization against more common strains is given to children annually in the UK (p149). Treatment is usually symptomatic. Antiviral agents may be considered in severe disease, or in at-risk children (e.g. chronic respiratory disease) presenting with milder illness during epidemics.

20.5   Lower respiratory tract

The bronchial tree and its blood supply are present by the 20th week of gestation, and thereafter only enlarge. In contrast, the alveoli increase in number from 20 million at birth to the adult complement of

300 million. Respiratory disease in early childhood may therefore interfere with future lung development and cause direct lung damage. Small airways obstruct or collapse early, leading to poor oxygenation or collapse of a lung segment.

20.5.1 Bronchitis

Acute bronchitis occurs at all ages and is characterized by cough, fever and often wheezing. It is a common feature of influenza and whooping cough. Persistent bacterial bronchitis is an occasional cause of chronic cough in children and may be confused with asthma. A cough swab may aid diagnosis, and a prolonged course of antibiotics (2 weeks or longer) is usually effective.

20.5.2 Bronchiolitis

Bronchiolitis is the most common cause of severe respiratory infection in infancy; 70% is due to RSV, and 90% of children are immune to this virus by 2 years of age. Most children remain at home with this infection, but 1–2% of all infants are admitted each year, usually during the winter epidemics.

Younger infants and those with marked respiratory distress are more likely to need hospital admission. Supportive management includes skilled nursing, intravenous fluids, nasogastric feeding and oxygen, usually monitored with pulse oximetry. Nasogastric feeding is needed frequently to maintain fluid and calorie intake. Antibiotics are usually not indicated unless there is evidence of bacterial infection or severe disease. The RSV may be detected by fluorescent antibody test on nasopharyngeal secretions. Most infants recover within a few days. Up to half of infants with RSV bronchiolitis subsequently develop recurrent wheezing.

20.5.3 Community-acquired pneumonia

This is most common in young children and in older children with a chronic condition affecting respiratory function (e.g. cystic fibrosis, severe cerebral palsy). A wide variety of organisms can be responsible. The child may appear ill with cough, fever and respiratory distress, but sometimes symptoms and signs are non-specific. Cyanosis occurs in severe cases and infants may develop cardiac failure. Focal signs of crepitations, decreased air entry and bronchial breathing may be present with lobar consolidation, and there may be a transient pleural rub, or sometimes an effusion.

> 🔑 Consider bacterial pneumonia if persistent or recurrent fever >38.5 °C in a child with chest recession and raised respiratory rate. If oxygen saturations are ≥92%, and the child is well enough to remain at home, they can be treated with oral antibiotics (e.g. amoxicillin), and no chest X-ray is needed.

In more unwell children seen in the hospital, a chest X-ray may be performed, especially if there is diagnostic doubt. It may show patchy or lobar consolidation (Figure 20.2). Oxygen is given if saturations <92% and a broad-spectrum antibiotic (e.g. oral amoxicillin), since it is difficult to differentiate bacterial from viral pneumonias. Intravenous antibiotics are given if the child cannot take or absorb oral, is septic or the pneumonia complicated (e.g. by effusion). In young children who cannot take oral feeds, consider nasogastric feeding (note the tube may compromise breathing), or intravenous fluids.

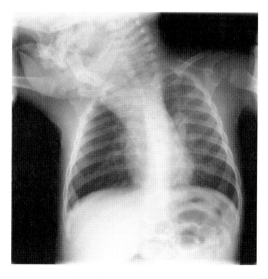

Figure 20.2 Chest X-ray showing right upper lobe collapse and consolidation.

> **Pneumonia: causative agents**
>
> - Common
>   - Viral (especially RSV)
>   - *Streptococcus pneumonia*
> - Uncommon
>   - *Mycoplasma pneumonia*
>   - *Staphylococcus aureus*
>   - *Mycobacterium tuberculosis*
>   - *Haemophilus influenzae* (rare since the introduction of Hib vaccine).

Lobar pneumonia is usually caused by *Streptococcus pneumoniae*, and penicillin achieves dramatic improvement within 24 h. In the ill child, the causative organism is not known initially and broad-spectrum antibiotics are used. Not all children are severely ill and some can be treated at home. Fluid intake is more important than food.

PRACTICE POINT

Remember that pneumonia may present with few respiratory symptoms or signs, and with 'non-respiratory' symptoms such as abdominal pain or vomiting. Therefore, a chest X-ray is often performed as part of the workup for a young, febrile, ill child where there is no obvious focus of infection.

If improvement does not occur, or if signs or symptoms are still present after a week, careful examination including chest X-ray should be repeated to exclude complications such as pleural effusion or lobar collapse. In the older child particularly, mycoplasma should be considered. The possibility of *tuberculosis* should never be forgotten.

Staphylococcal pneumonia is a severe form of lung infection which usually affects young children and those with chronic predisposing disease. It is characterized by lung cysts on X-ray and the sudden appearance of empyema or pneumothorax. Prolonged treatment is required with an anti-staphylococcal antibiotic.

20.5.4 Inhaled foreign bodies

Toddlers are most at risk because they tend to put everything into their mouths. Older children sometimes accidentally inhale objects during games or whilst stuffing their mouths too full of peanuts or sweets. A foreign body may lodge at any level. At the time, the child will cough, splutter or make choking noises, but the episode is quickly forgotten and may not come out in the history without specific questioning.

PRACTICE POINT

Ask about foreign body inhalation when persistent cough, or chest infection not resolving.

In the larynx, an object is likely to cause a croupy cough and stridor. If it passes through the larynx, it will lodge in a bronchus (right middle lobe or a lower lobe most often) and there will be no symptoms for a few days until infection, collapse or obstructive emphysema develop.

If a foreign body is suspected, radiography may demonstrate it (if it is radio-opaque) or show associated changes. Diagnosis may require direct laryngoscopy and bronchoscopy, which will be required to remove the object.

20.6 The wheezy child

Wheezing is an obstructive respiratory sound arising in the smaller branches of the bronchial tree: on auscultation, rhonchi can be heard. They are most marked in expiration because the bronchial tree dilates in inspiration.

Wheezing is most common in young infants, when it is usually triggered by viral infections, and diagnosed as 'viral-induced wheeze'. Some children have recurrent episodes limited to the first 2 years. In others, recurrent bouts of wheezing are the prelude to a diagnosis of asthma.

 Recurrent wheeze occurs in over 10% of children. The prevalence of mild and moderate asthma has increased.

20.7 Asthma

Asthma is one of the family of conditions grouped together under the term 'atopy'. The others include eczema and hay fever. All have raised IgE levels as part of the underlying pathology. It has a strong genetic basis, and it is unusual to make a diagnosis of asthma where there is no history of atopic conditions in either the child or the family.

 Asthma

Recurrent, reversible obstruction of the small airways

Key symptoms are *episodic* and *clusters* of several:

- Cough
- Shortness of breath
- Wheeze
- Chest tightness
- Exercise induced.

It is important to try to understand the underlying factors in each wheezy child if the best help is to be given. In young children, URTIs appear to be the most common precipitating factor, but as the child grows up others may become apparent: specific allergens, exercise, emotional upsets and changes of weather or environment (Figure 20.3).

 RESOURCE

The Scottish Intercollegiate Guideline Network (SIGN) website (**www.sign.ac.uk**) has a joint asthma guideline written with the British Thoracic Society (SIGN guideline 158). A free smartphone app is available for SIGN guidelines.

20.7.1   Asthma diagnosis

Diagnosis can be difficult in young children, who frequently have the alternative diagnosis of viral-induced wheeze. After thorough assessment, you should record the probability as high, intermediate or low based on the following factors:

Where there is diagnostic doubt in older children, the following may be helpful: spirometry; peak flow charting; reversibility after bronchodilator; challenge tests; and tests for eosinophilic inflammation or atopy. In younger children, response (or not) to treatment may be helpful in diagnosis.

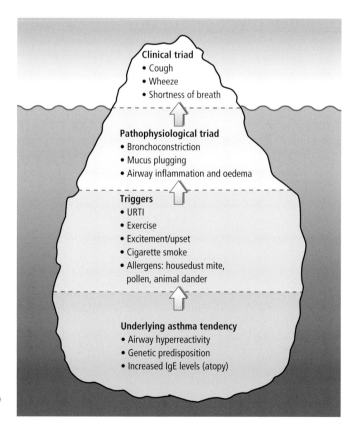

Figure 20.3 The pathogenesis of asthma. The clinical symptoms are the visible tip of an aetiological iceberg.

Increased probability of asthma	Decreased probability of asthma
• Episodic symptoms: cough, shortness of breath (including chest tightness) and wheeze • Diurnal variation, e.g. worse at night • Worse following exposure to asthma triggers (see box) • Personal or family history of atopy • Wheeze confirmed on auscultation by health professional • Improvement with asthma treatment • No pointers to alternative diagnoses	• Symptoms with colds only, no interval symptoms • Isolated cough • Symptoms suggesting hyperventilation (e.g. peripheral tingling) • Chest examination repeatedly normal when symptomatic • Normal PEFR or spirometry when symptomatic • No response to trial of asthma treatment • Clinical features pointing to alternative diagnosis (Table 20.3)

Common asthma triggers

Infection
Viral infection is a common precipitant of asthma: infection is likely to be important in children who have most trouble in winter.

Allergy
Allergens can be best identified from the history (e.g. after specific exposure or in the pollen season). A family history of allergies is common. Specific antibody tests add little to management.

Emotions
Exceptionally, a severe emotional upset may precipitate a first attack of wheezing. Commonly, excitement or anxiety can precipitate or aggravate attacks.

Exercise
Exercise-induced wheezing occurs most readily when running in a cold atmosphere. Beware the child who can begin a game of football but not last longer than 20 min. Many asthmatics become wheezy on exertion, especially if it involves running.

Atmosphere
Dusty air, 'stuffy' and smoke-filled rooms, or changes in air temperature may precipitate wheezing.

 PRACTICE POINTS

Clarify what the parents mean by 'wheeze' – they may mean something different.

Wheeze heard on auscultation by a health professional is important in diagnosis – ensure this is recorded clearly.

20.7.2 Assessing severity of asthma (Table 20.4)

Table 20.4 **History, examination and investigation of asthma**

History	Examination	Investigation
Acute		
What do child/parents think?	Level of respiratory distress	Oxygen saturation
Therapy received	Tachycardia	Blood gas – abnormalities occur late
Can child run/walk/drink/talk?	Altered conscious level (drowsy or irritable)	Chest X-ray – if severe
	Beware silent chest (↓ air entry in severe attack)	PEFR – unreliable in acute attack
Chronic		
Child/parent opinion	Growth	Serial PEFR
Current therapy	Chest shape	Spirometry
Hospital admission	– ↑ AP diameter	
Lifestyle changes	– Harrison's sulci (p39)	
Sport		
School attendance		

20.7.3 Management

The aim is to reduce the frequency and severity of attacks and to give the child and family confidence that they can cope with attacks without disruption of home or school life. Precipitating factors should be sought.

RESOURCE   Asthma management plans

Supporting self/parent management improves outcomes: provide a personalized written plan, with a clear summary of current treatment and advice about what to do in an exacerbation – this can be combined with a symptom diary (with peak flows for older children). For a good example of a plan, go to **www.asthma.org. uk** and search 'child's asthma action plan'.

Those at home are advised not to smoke. Emotional problems at home or school can often be helped, but asthma can generate its own emotional problems for the family. It can be a frightening condition.

In some children, the history of asthma is obvious. In others, colds 'go to the chest', cough persists and the parents may not notice the wheezing. Typically, the asthmatic child will have recurrent respiratory infections which last longer than those of her siblings. Nighttime symptoms of poor sleeping or cough should raise suspicions. It is so common that it should always be sought on direct inquiry in every paediatric history.

20.7.3.1 Peak expiratory flow rate (PEFR or 'Peak flow')

Normal peak expiratory flow rate is related to height, not age – you will find charts in outpatient clinics and wards.

PEFR = {(height above 100 cm) × 5 + 100} ± 100 L/min (Figure 20.4)
Children from about 6 years old can do peak flows, with training and practice.

PRACTICE POINT

Doing a peak flow measurement (Figure 20.5)
- Ask the child to stand.
- Use a new or sterilized mouthpiece in the meter.
- Demonstrate use: 'Don't block meter indicator with finger, take a deep breath, lips around the mouthpiece, blow hard and fast.'
- Take the best of three readings.
- Interpret from chart (or according to personal best)
- A peak flow diary (where the readings are charted daily on a graph) is helpful in guiding management.

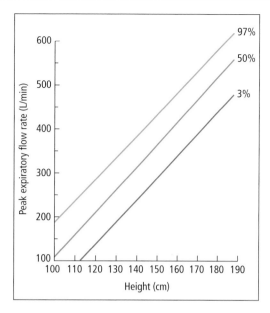

Figure 20.4 Normal peak expiratory flow rate and height.

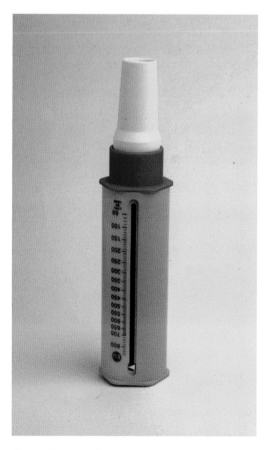

Figure 20.5 Peak flow meter.

TREATMENT **Making sense of peak flow readings**

Work from their 'personal best' when asthma well-controlled, otherwise derive from the chart.
The 80/60/40 rule:

- below 80% – asthma is worse – take bronchodilator 4 hourly, urgent medical review if doesn't last 4 h or not better in 24 h; consider oral steroids;
- below 60% is an asthma attack – call for help, take bronchodilator 1 puff every 30–60 s up to 10 puffs, call for urgent help if not improving
- below 40% is potentially life-threatening attack, call for urgent help.

PRACTICE POINT **Management when diagnosis uncertain**

(intermediate or low probability)
Consider:

- PEFR/spirometry before and after bronchodilators
- Trial of very low or low-dose inhaled corticosteroids with symptom diary
- Further investigation
- Specialist referral.

20.7.3.2 Administration of therapy

Whenever possible, asthma therapy should be given by inhalation (Figures 20.6 and 20.7). In children of school age, dry powder inhalers or metered dose aerosol inhalers (MDI) with a spacer device may be used. All aerosol agents are more effective through a spacer device (Figure 20.8), avoiding the need to

synchronize inhalation with the aerosol and improving distribution of the drug in the bronchial tree. In infants, a metered dose inhaler with spacer device fitted with a face mask may be used with instruction. Nebulized therapy can be given with a little cooperation on the part of the child. It is always best to ask the parent or child to hold the face mask. This is particularly valuable during acute attacks requiring oxygen to deliver bronchodilators (see also Figure 29.2).

Oral therapy with salbutamol or terbutaline is not effective, and side effects are more likely. Leukotriene receptor antagonists (LTRAs) can be given orally as granules sprinkled on food or as chewable tablets, and so can be useful in younger children. Long-acting bronchodilators can be combined with low-dose steroids in a single inhaler to simplify treatment. Occasionally, oral steroids and xanthines (e.g. theophylline) are necessary in children with severe chronic disease (under specialist care). Oral prednisolone may be given in a short course over a few days to bring about resolution of an acute severe attack.

The most common reason for poor control in chronic asthma is not adhering to treatment – discuss this regularly at reviews, and look for practical ways to assist. If control deteriorates abruptly, make sure the family have not just acquired a pet.

Early, adequate prophylaxis may reduce the likelihood of later, severe disease.

🔑 Annual deaths from childhood asthma have gradually fallen from a peak in the 1960s, but 20–30 children die each year in the UK. This compares to over 1300 deaths annually in adults, the vast majority in over-65s.

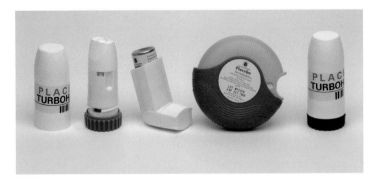

Figure 20.6 Inhalers used for asthma. The central one is a metered dose aerosol inhaler; the round one is an Accuhaler (a dry powder device); the others are Turbohalers (also dry powder devices).

Mutation analysis is extremely helpful but cannot exclude CF as not all mutations are known. In affected families, it forms a reliable test for foetal and neonatal screening. Pancreatic damage results in raised serum immune-reactive trypsin in the first 6 weeks of life. This can be detected in the blood spots collected for routine neonatal screening and is now part of the national UK neonatal screening programme. High sensitivity but relatively low specificity means that the test will pick up children without the disease, leaving parents worried until they discover that their child does not have CF. Pre-symptomatic diagnosis, however, allows early introduction of the modern aggressive therapy which has transformed the prognosis.

20.8.3 Treatment and prognosis

The respiratory problems of CF are progressive. In the 1960s, babies survived for only a few months or years. Modern aggressive therapy, started at an early age, has transformed the prognosis for CF (Table 20.5, Figure 20.13). Median life expectancy is now mid-40s,

Table 20.5 **Treatment of cystic fibrosis**		
Respiratory	**Nutritional**	**Family**
Physiotherapy at least twice every day	Constant monitoring	Education
Early anti-staphylococcal prophylaxis	Dietetic supervision	Teach parents/child to do physiotherapy
Aggressive intravenous high-dose antibiotics for exacerbations	High energy/protein 150% of average requirements	Recognition of relapse
Bronchodilators	High-fat diet	Home intravenous antibiotics
DNAse to reduce viscosity of secretions	Pancreatic therapy enzyme replacement	Genetic counselling
Avoid cross-infection		Financial help (e.g. Disability Living Allowance)
Precision medicines targeting CFTR function		Emotional support

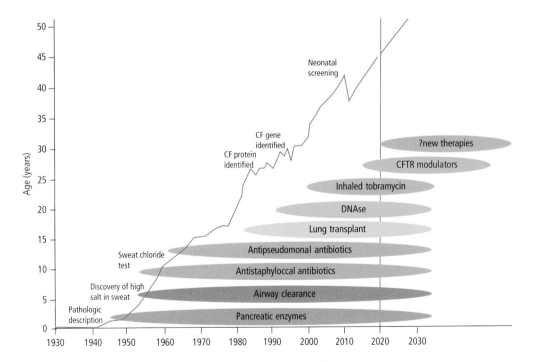

Figure 20.13 Advances in cystic fibrosis treatment. Figure shows median life expectancy over time. Latest advances include CFTR modulator treatments which aim to get the CFTR channel to the cell membrane or improve its function. *Source:* Adapted from the Cystic Fibrosis Trust (www.cysticfibrosis.org.uk) with permission.

and most can live reasonably normal and productive lives. Treatment is best provided by multidisciplinary teams working in specialist centres. Adherence to the demanding treatment regime can difficult. Lung transplant is sometime possible. New treatments targeting the CFTR protein may be transformative for many patients, depending on their exact gene mutation. Gene therapy is an exciting future possibility.

for admission, and you need to know these conditions well. Make sure that you are familiar with asthma treatment. Cystic fibrosis, although rarer, illustrates the challenges of managing a chronic condition in childhood. The transformation in prognosis over recent decades is gratifying, but treatment is not easy.

Research Trail

Cystic fibrosis outcomes have steadily improved through incremental research-based additions to treatment (Figure 20.13). Discovery of the ΔF508 mutation in the CFTR gene in the late 1980s is now leading to personalized treatments that modulate CFTR function.

Next Research Trail on page 311

FOR YOUR LOG

- Observe a nasopharyngeal aspirate being taken (for RSV in bronchiolitis)
- Watch a child's inhaler technique being checked.
- Measure a child's peak expiratory flow and know how to interpret it.
- Be familiar with asthma treatment devices (inhalers, aerochambers, nebulizers)
- Observe a sweat test.

PRACTICE POINT   Long-term complications of CF

- Respiratory failure
- Psychological/emotional problems
- Diabetes mellitus
- Portal hypertension
- Hepatic cirrhosis
- Cor pulmonale
- Distal intestinal obstruction syndrome
- Male infertility.

OSCE TIP

- Child with chronic respiratory problem, e.g. CF, asthma (see OSCE station 20.2).
- Acute respiratory illness – so common a child may have some wheeze.
- Assessment of acute or long-term respiratory status.
- Chest X-ray, e.g. pneumonia, pneumothorax.
- Video of severe asthma attack.
- Explain use of inhalers, peak flow meter and chart.

Summary

Respiratory problems, particularly bronchiolitis, croup, pneumonia and asthma, are common reasons

See EMQ 20.1, EMQ 20.2 and EMQ 20.3 at the end of the book.

OSCE station 20.1: Examination of the respiratory system

Clinical approach:

Check hands
- Clubbing
- Colour
- Perfusion

Check face
- Colour
- Anaemia
- Respiratory distress

Chest

Inspection
Acute signs
- Respiratory rate
- Recession/increased work of breathing
- Added noises (cough, wheeze, etc.)

Chronic signs
- Chest shape
- Pectus carinatum/AP diameter
- Harrison's sulci

Percussion
- Percuss upper, mid and lower zones, anteriorly and posteriorly
- Dullness over the heart is normal

Auscultation
- Added noises
  - Stridor
  - Wheeze
  - Crackles
  - Crepitation
  - Rub

James is 14 years old. Please examine his respiratory system

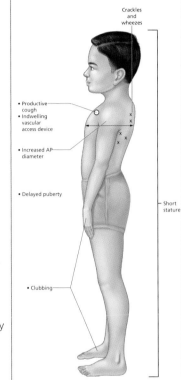

Crackles and wheezes

- Productive cough
- Indwelling vascular access device
- Increased AP diameter
- Delayed puberty
- Clubbing

Short stature

James has cystic fibrosis with signs of chronic lung infection and asthma. He has poor growth and no signs of puberty.

Never forget:
- Say hello and introduce yourself
- General health
- Colour – ?pale/?cyanosed
- Quickly assess growth, nutrition and development
- Mention the obvious (e.g. drip, leg in plaster)

Look around for:
- Inhalers
- Sputum pot
- Nasogastric tube, gastrostomy
- Vascular access device
- Oxygen – mask, nasal prongs
- Medications

Special points
- Evidence of atopic disease (e.g. eczema)
- Beware transmitted noises; listen again after asking the child to cough
- Percussion is usually unhelpful in children under 2 years, and they don't like it; omit it and explain why
- Percuss onto your finger, not direct onto clavicle
- Downward displacement of the liver occurs if the chest is overexpanded

OSCE station 20.2: Prescribing and explaining asthma treatment

This station assesses the candidate's ability to prescribe, explain and demonstrate appropriate asthma treatment.

'You are an FY1 doctor attached to a paediatric ward. Abigail is a 4-year-old girl admitted with asthma, who needs medications to be prescribed before going home. You have been asked to prescribe them and explain their use to the parent. You have been told by the registrar that she needs to be on a regular preventer inhaler at a standard dose, and a reliever inhaler. She needs two more days of oral steroids at a dose of 2 mg per kg per day. Her weight is 15 kg.'

You have been asked to

- Prescribe the medication
- Explain to the parent how and when to use it.

(continued on next page)

(continued)

You have 10 min for this station.

(A standard discharge prescription sheet, and demonstration inhalers, etc., would be provided.)

Simulated patient script

You are Jane/Richard Riley and you are the parent of 4-year-old Abigail who has about to go home from the paediatric ward. You have been told she has asthma, and this has been explained to you. Now one of the junior doctors is going to come and explain about the asthma treatment Abigail will be starting.

- Abigail was diagnosed with asthma on this admission having had four episodes of being wheezy and short of breath in the past 2 months. She had not been admitted until this episode.
- If asked what you know about asthma, say that someone has explained to you about what asthma is, and you just need to know how to use the medications.
- If asked what you know about using an inhaler, say 'Well I have been told that the inhaler will help Abigail's breathing but that's all.'
- The candidate should give you details of drugs to be used but, if he/she does not ask, say 'What do I use it with?'
- Follow the candidate's instructions as you understand them.

This is a 10-min station. The candidate is a junior doctor (FY1), who is asked to explain how and when to use the medication and demonstrate the use of a metered dose inhaler (MDI) and spacer – the standard device for the treatment of asthma.

You will be asked to mark the candidate on 2 points:
- I understood how to use the inhalers
- I understood when to use each inhaler

Marksheet

Prescription
- Beclomethasone MDI 200 µg bd inh via aerochamber (100 bd acceptable)
- Salbutamol MDI 200–600 (2–6 puffs) prn inh via aerochamber
- Prednisolone 30 mg (6 tablets) daily for 2 days
- One aerochamber
- Clearly written, signed and dated

Introduction
- Introduction and orientation (name and role, explains purpose of interview, confirms patient's agreement)
- Elicits parent's knowledge of device
- Names the device
- Explains purpose of device
- Explains clinical situation when it is used

Inhaler technique: teaches/shows
- Shake canister
- Correctly attach to aerochamber
- Ensure mask is over nose and mouth and make a seal with the face
- Breathe out fully
- Spray 1 puff
- Hold mask on and allow the child to breathe normally for 10 s
- Wait 30 seconds to see if repeat dose is needed (for bronchodilators)
- Shake canister and repeat dose

Use of inhaler:
- Explains which drugs should be used
- Explains how the drugs should be used
- Rapport (shows interest, respect and concern, appropriate body language
- Information giving and explaining (clear, unambiguous explanation, jargon-free, well paced, checks understanding, invites questions
- Fluency and organization (systemic and logical flow)
- Closure (summarizes main points, thanks parent)

SP to mark:
- I understood how to use the inhalers
- I understood when to use each inhaler.

21.4 Neonatal presentations

PRACTICE POINT

If a newborn with a heart murmur is fit to go home, tell the parents what symptoms may occur. Their baby needs to come back early if they are concerned.

21.4.1 Heart murmur

The most common clinical presentation is the discovery of a heart murmur during routine examination in the first days of life (Section 8.4.1). Perform a full clinical assessment and a careful search for other congenital abnormalities. If any cardiac symptoms are present, arrange urgent cardiological assessment. If the infant remains well, but the murmur persists beyond 24–48 h, assessment by an experienced paediatrician or cardiologist is justified. In most paediatric practice, if a murmur is present over the first weeks of life, even if it is thought to be innocent, echocardiography is performed.

21.4.2 Cyanosis

Distinguish between central and peripheral cyanosis.

PRACTICE POINT

Central
- Tongue and peripheries blue
- Concentration of deoxygenated haemoglobin >5 g/dL
- Indicates significant disease

Peripheral
- Hands and feet blue
- Common and normal in the first days of life.

In some infants, cyanosis becomes gradually more apparent, while the infant remains otherwise well. This presentation is typical of Fallot tetralogy (see Section 21.5.4.1). In some infants, the presentation is dramatic. The infant is hypoxic and may be collapsed and acidotic, with a clinical picture which is hard to distinguish from severe infection. A nitrogen washout test may be helpful. The infant is placed in 100% - for

10–20 min. In severe lung disease, persistent foetal circulation and cyanotic congenital heart disease, the blood oxygen does not rise.

In some conditions, blood flow to the lungs is dependent on the patent ductus arteriosus (PDA). The infant becomes very ill when the ductus closes. The emergency treatment aims to maintain duct patency with prostaglandin. Neonatal intensive care and ventilation are often required. Definitive treatment depends upon diagnosis.

21.4.3 Heart failure

Acute heart failure may occur in left-sided obstructive lesions (e.g. coarctation of the aorta). In such infants, systemic blood flow may depend upon the ductus, and prostaglandin may be used. Over the first weeks of life, increasing left-to-right shunting may produce right heart failure of insidious onset with a characteristic set of signs and symptoms (see Section 21.7). In mild failure, these are hard to recognize.

21.5 Classification of congenital heart disease

Eight lesions represent 80% of congenital heart disease (Figure 21.2). Obstructive lesions reduce flow in the outflow tracts or aorta. If the lesion produces a connection between the systemic and pulmonary

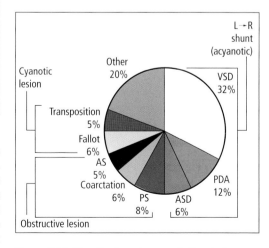

Figure 21.2 Classification of congenital heart disease.

circulations, a left-to-right shunt occurs. In the cyanotic lesions, there is obstruction to the pulmonary circulation (e.g. Fallot) or abnormal circulation (e.g. transposition of the great arteries).

21.5.1   Diagnosis

Initially, assessment is by clinical examination. Chest X-ray and ECG are helpful, but the most important diagnostic tool is echocardiography with Doppler assessment, which allows estimation of flow. Only rarely is cardiac catheterization required. Full assessment of non-cardiac problems can be critically important, if major surgery is being considered.

21.5.2   Left-to-right shunts

21.5.2.1   Ventricular septal defect (VSD) (Figure 21.3)

The natural history of VSD depends upon the size of the defect, the changes that occur with growth and the pulmonary vascular resistance.

Small defects

Patients have no symptoms, and the heart murmur is heard during routine examination. Seventy-five per cent close in the first 10 years of life (the majority by two years) but closure goes on occurring in adult life. The only risk is of bacterial endocarditis.

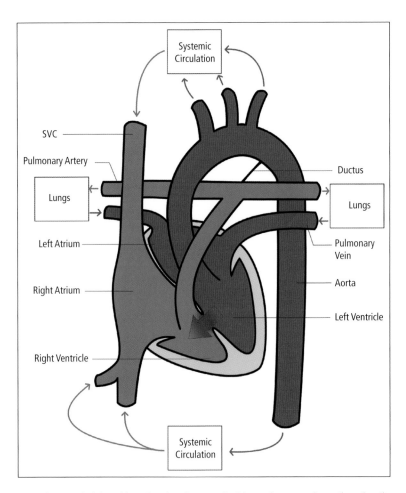

Figure 21.3 Ventricular septal defect. Note that the diagrams in this section are schematic rather than anatomical and provide a simple approach to understanding the various lesions. Oxygenated blood is shown in red, deoxygenated blood in blue.

Medium-sized defects

These cause symptoms in infancy. Heart failure results in poor feeding and slow weight gain. Symptoms appear in the first months of life, often precipitated by a chest infection. Improvement occurs following medical treatment. As the child grows, the defect becomes relatively smaller, symptoms lessen and weight gain improves. Spontaneous closure usually occurs.

Large defects

Symptoms begin in the first weeks of life. Heart failure is difficult to control, and tube feeding is necessary. A small number close, but most need surgery. In infancy, persistent high pulmonary blood flow leads to increased pulmonary vascular resistance. The volume of the left-to-right shunt diminishes and heart failure improves. It is important not to be misled by this apparent improvement because, if the defect is not closed before the age of two years, changes in the lung vessels become permanent. Without surgery, pulmonary vascular disease worsens, the shunt reverses, the patient becomes cyanosed and breathless and life expectancy is markedly reduced (Eisenmenger syndrome). The only management of pulmonary vascular disease is prevention with early surgery.

Signs

- Pan-systolic murmur at the left sternal edge (turbulent L → R blood flow)
- Maximal in the third and fourth left interspaces
- Loud murmurs cause a systolic thrill
- Murmur is harsh, like the sound of wood being sawn
- Murmur may become louder as the lesion closes, because of greater turbulence.

Treatment

- Control the heart failure with medical treatment (e.g. diuretics, angiotensin-converting enzyme (ACE) inhibitors)
- Surgical closure (cardiopulmonary bypass) if symptoms cannot be controlled or danger of pulmonary vascular disease.

21.5.2.2 Patent ductus arteriosus (PDA) (see Figure 9.4)

PDA is most common in the preterm infant. Murmur and heart failure are noted in the first weeks during intensive care, and it may be difficult to reduce the infant's ventilation requirements. Control of heart failure may be sufficient. Some preterm infants require duct closure medically, using indomethacin as a prostaglandin inhibitor, or by surgical ligation. Spontaneous closure occurs up to three months after birth.

In the term infant, if the ductus is patent during the first two weeks of life, spontaneous closure is rare. A large PDA leads to heart failure, and in others, the persisting risk of bacterial endocarditis is an indication for surgical closure.

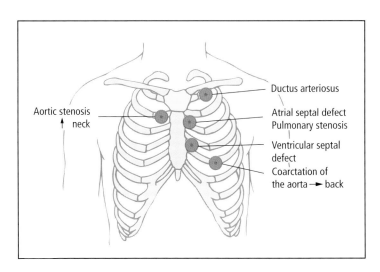

Aortic stenosis
↑ neck

Ductus arteriosus

Atrial septal defect
Pulmonary stenosis

Ventricular septal defect

Coarctation of the aorta → back

Figure 21.4 The mumur is heard loudest at the point shown. Some loud murmurs can be heard over the whole precordium. Some murmurs radiate in a characteristic direction.

Signs

- Collapsing pulses due to sudden leak of blood from the aorta to the pulmonary artery
- Preterm infant may have tachycardia and bounding pulses
- Continuous, 'machinery' (systolic and diastolic) murmur
- Maximal under left clavicle (Figure 21.4)
- May be a thrill.

Treatment

- Treat heart failure medically
- If duct persists, close by surgical ligation or using small 'double umbrella' device placed in the ductus through a cardiac catheter.

21.5.2.3 Atrial septal defect (ASD)

(Figure 21.5)

ASD does not usually cause symptoms in childhood because the left-to-right shunt is small. In the majority, a heart murmur is discovered during routine examination and the child has few or no symptoms. Symptoms occur in the second and third decades, pulmonary hypertension develops secondary to the large blood flow into the lungs, and heart failure and atrial dysrhythmias result.

Signs

- Right ventricular heave – increased blood volume
- Ejection systolic murmur in pulmonary area – excessive blood flow through a normal pulmonary valve

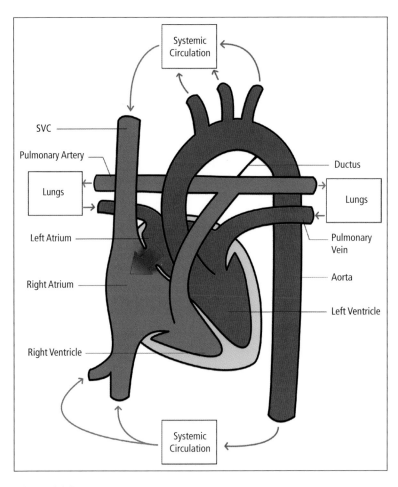

Figure 21.5 Atrial septal defect.

- Deoxygenated systemic venous blood → aorta
- Mixing of two circulations depends on one of:
  - Atrial septum
  - Ductus arteriosus
  - VSD.

Signs

- There must be a connection between the two parallel circulations to allow some mixing, or the condition is incompatible with life
- Presents acutely in the first days of life, as the ductus arteriosus closes and cyanosis increases
- Child becomes breathless, unable to feed and may be extremely ill
- May or may not be a murmur.

X-ray

The heart has a narrow pedicle and is like an egg, with the pointed part of the egg forming the apex of the heart ('egg on its side').

Treatment

- Without urgent treatment, these children die.
- Prostaglandin is given to maintain patency of the ductus arteriosus.
- Emergency treatment is balloon septostomy. A cardiac catheter is passed through the atrial septum. A balloon on the end is then inflated and pulled back sharply into the right atrium in order to tear the atrial septum. This allows mixing of blood between the two atria.
- Surgical correction is performed in the first months of life by 'arterial switch', when the aorta and pulmonary artery are divided above the valves and switched over.

21.6 Surgical treatment of congenital heart disease

As cardiac surgery advances, there is a tendency to operate on the common lesions earlier in life. This often means operating before the child has any symptoms. Surgery is generally safe, with operative mortality less than 5%. In a large majority, long-term myocardial function is normal.

PRACTICE POINT **Informing parents about heart disease**

- Parents are shocked to hear their child has heart disease
- Cause is usually unknown – it is not their fault
- Congenital heart disease is not like ischaemic heart disease
- Exercise restriction is hardly ever necessary (except in severe AS)
- Try to provide written information and a diagram
- Echocardiography (cardiac ultrasound) is an important early investigation
- Not all congenital heart disease requires surgery
- Advice about endocarditis is important.

21.7 Cardiac failure

Heart failure is a medical emergency. It occurs more commonly in the first three months of life than in any other period of childhood and is usually due to congenital heart disease (Figure 21.10). Earlier onset implies a more severe heart lesion. It is also caused by myocarditis, endocarditis and dysrhythmias.

Clinical features

- Poor feeding
- Breathless on exertion
- Sweating
- Poor weight gain
- Excess weight gain (oedema).

21.7.1 Treatment

- Prompt treatment is essential
- Cardiac assessment (echo, chest X-ray, ECG) and treatment of cause
- Prop the child up and give oxygen
- Correct acidosis, hypoglycaemia, hypocalcaemia or anaemia
- Treat respiratory infection with antibiotics
- Feed by nasogastric tube
- Medication: diuretics are important; furosemide is often combined with spironolactone to prevent

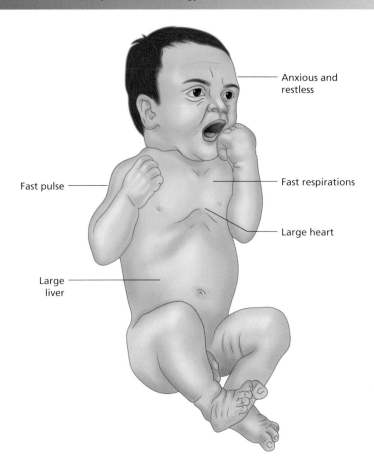

Anxious and restless

Fast pulse

Fast respirations

Large heart

Large liver

Figure 21.10 Cardiac failure in infancy.

potassium loss. Systemic vascular resistance and the work of the left ventricle can be reduced with a vasodilator (e.g. ACE inhibitor).

21.8 Dysrhythmias

Abnormalities of sinus rhythm are not usually of cardiac origin. Bradycardia is often associated with hypoxia. A tachycardia is often seen in association with fever, dehydration or any acute illness. If episodic dysrhythmia is suspected from the history, ambulatory 24 h ECG monitoring can be extremely helpful.

21.8.1 Supraventricular tachycardia (SVT)

SVT is the most common symptomatic dysrhythmia in childhood. It may rarely occur in utero and is controlled by treating the mother. Infants with SVT become acutely ill, collapsed and grey, and need urgent help. The pulse is very fast, too fast to count. ECG shows a narrow complex tachycardia (greater than 250 bpm).

21.8.1.1 Treatment

- Oxygen
- Vagal stimulation (facial immersion in iced water or the application of an ice bag) if well
- Rapid intravenous injection of adenosine is usually successful
- If unstable with depressed conscious level, perform synchronized cardioversion
- Intensive care may be required
- Some children require long-term treatment to prevent recurrence.

21.8.2 Ventricular extrasystoles

In childhood, extrasystoles are not uncommon and usually of no significance. If there are symptoms or

22.1.2 Abdominal pain

22.1.2.1 Acute abdominal pain

Abdominal pain

Condition	Site of pain and tenderness
Non-organic pain	Central
URTI/tonsillitis	Central/RIF
Pyelonephritis	Loins
Lower lobe pneumonia	Upper abdomen
Constipation	Lower abdomen
Mesenteric adenitis	Lower abdomen, often RIF
Pancreatitis	Central/may radiate to back

RIF, right iliac fossa; URTI, upper respiratory tract infection.

This important symptom is highly non-specific. Acute central abdominal pain and vomiting are, for example, common symptoms of tonsillitis. In infants, abdominal pain may be inferred from spasms of crying, restlessness and drawing up the knees. Children can indicate the site of a pain from about the age of 2 years. If there is generalized illness, vomiting, bowel disturbance or fever assess carefully and re-examine after a few hours. Intussusception, complicated hernia and appendicitis are amongst the important surgical causes. Acute abdominal pain is a typical presenting feature in diabetic ketoacidosis (Section 28.1), Henoch–Schönlein syndrome (Section 24.3.5) and sickle cell disease (Section 26.2.2.3).

Appendicitis

Acute appendicitis occurs at all ages but is uncommon under the age of 2 years. The classical history of central abdominal pain, moving to the right iliac fossa, aggravated by movement and associated with fever and acute phase response, raises suspicion, which may be confirmed by the finding of localized tenderness in the right iliac fossa. Unfortunately, it is not always that easy.

Diagnostic difficulties may be caused by an appendix in an unusual position. Diagnosis of appendicitis is particularly difficult in younger children. The doctor who diagnoses appendicitis before perforation in a 2-year-old deserves praise. Consider imaging (ultrasound/CT) in difficult cases.

22.1.2.2 Chronic abdominal pain

 PRACTICE POINT

Protracted gastrointestinal symptoms: if examination and growth are normal, serious pathology is unlikely.

Recurrent abdominal pain is common throughout childhood and usually of no serious significance when the child is otherwise healthy (Figure 22.2). History, examination, growth assessment and urine microscopy and culture are always justified. The idea that one should exclude all organic causes is naive and usually not possible. Constipation is a common cause and is usually, but not always, apparent on history and examination.

In some children, recurrent abdominal pain betrays emotional disorders. It has often persisted for a year or more by the time medical advice is sought. The child may complain of pain several times in a week and then not at all for a month or two. As children with recurrent abdominal pain are usually of school age, the parents often suspect some stress at school. In many there is a family history of irritable bowel syndrome or migraine, and the childhood equivalent of irritable bowel syndrome is increasingly well recognized. Irritable bowel syndrome, non-ulcer dyspepsia and abdominal migraine may be helped by specific treatments for these conditions.

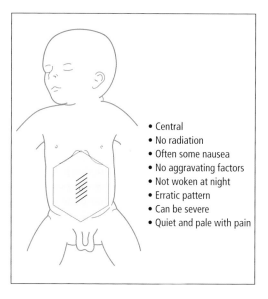

- Central
- No radiation
- Often some nausea
- No aggravating factors
- Not woken at night
- Erratic pattern
- Can be severe
- Quiet and pale with pain

Figure 22.2 Recurrent abdominal pain.

Recurrent abdominal pain

Features implying organic disease:
Pain
- Not central
- Wakes at night
- Related to food

Associated symptoms
- Vomiting/diarrhoea
- Generalized illness
- Dysuria, daytime enuresis

Growth failure.

22.1.3 Abdominal distension

Abdominal distension can be difficult to assess because of the great, normal variation. Toddlers are normally rather pot-bellied in comparison with older children. Causes include fat, faeces, flatus and fluid: do not forget to test for ascites (Section 3.5.5, p. 41).

PRACTICE POINT

The best test for abdominal distension – ask the mother 'Is it distended?'!

22.1.4 Diarrhoea

Diarrhoea or constipation requires detailed enquiry. The number and consistency of stools passed by children, especially infants, is very variable. Breast-fed babies pass loose, bright yellow stools, between seven times a day and once every 7 days. Bottle-fed babies pass paler, firmer stools which may cause straining

---

Causes of diarrhoea

Feeding errors
- In infants, too much, too little or the wrong kind
- In older children, dietary indiscretion

Inflammatory
- Bacterial or viral infection
- Postenteritic syndrome
- Ulcerative colitis/Crohn disease
- Giardiasis
- Parenteral infections

Malabsorption states
- Steatorrhoea (e.g. coeliac disease, cystic fibrosis[CF])
- Disaccharide intolerance

Food intolerance/allergy

Protein-losing enteropathy.

---

during defaecation. Unless this straining causes pain or rectal bleeding, it should not be called constipation.

Many toddlers and some older children continue to have three or four bowel actions a day, after meals. '*Toddler diarrhoea*' describes the occurrence of frequent loose stools at this age without any pathology and is due to a rapid bowel transit time. Undigested food is seen in the stool within a few hours of being eaten (our personal best was carrots at 20 min).

Overflow soiling in infants or children with chronic constipation and faecal impaction may be mistaken for diarrhoea.

22.1.5 Constipation and soiling

Chronic or severe constipation may lead to abdominal pain, abdominal distension, rectal bleeding and feeding problems, and may be associated with emotional and behaviour disorders (Section 12.5.2.1, p. 22).

Constipation is most common at 5–10 years. Often there is no obvious trigger, or there has been minor change in diet or bowel habit (for example with illness or travel). Hard stool causes pain or anal fissure which inhibits defaecation and increases constipation. At other times, poor toilet training has resulted in infrequent and incomplete bowel actions. The rectum becomes distended with impacted faeces. In extreme cases, only liquid matter can escape, causing overflow diarrhoea with faecal soiling (Figure 22.3). The child is often unaware of this.

TREATMENT   Management of constipation

General advice
- Increased dietary fibre (e.g. bran)
- Ideally the whole family should adopt a high-fibre diet
- Increased fluid and exercise
- Instant success is not to be expected – rectum takes time to resume its normal calibre and sensation

Bowel training
- Regular toileting (1–2 times daily, 20 minutes after meal – to benefit from the gastrocolic reflex)
- Can combine with star chart)

Laxatives
- Consider disimpaction – thorough emptying of accumulated faeces with laxatives (rarely enemas)
- Faecal softening agents (e.g. Macrogols – polyethylene glycol 3350 with electrolytes; lactulose)
- Stimulant laxative may be added later
- May be needed for many months.

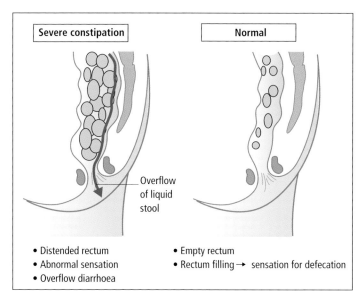

Severe constipation	Normal

Overflow of liquid stool

- Distended rectum
- Abnormal sensation
- Overflow diarrhoea

- Empty rectum
- Rectum filling → sensation for defecation

Figure 22.3 Constipation and overflow.

The abdomen contains hard, faecal masses, often filling the lower half of the abdomen. There is unlikely to be confusion with the rare Hirschsprung disease (see Section 22.2.2.1, p. 252), which usually presents at a much earlier age with failure to thrive.

RESOURCE

Go to **www.nice.org.uk** and search for 'constipation in children' to review the latest UK NICE guidance. Also see OSCE station 22.2: Constipation.

Encopresis (deliberate deposition of stool in inappropriate places) is a symptom of serious psychological upset, and the advice of a child psychiatrist should be sought.

22.1.6   Rectal bleeding

Blood in the stools is an alarming symptom, although the cause is often trivial. The most common cause is an anal fissure. Bleeding from the duodenum or above will usually cause melaena, although copious bleeding (e.g. swallowed blood after epistaxis or tonsillectomy) may cause red blood to appear with the stool. Blood from the ileum or colon is freely mixed with faecal matter; that from the rectum or anus is only on the surface of the stool. Examination of the perineum, anus and rectal examination (Section 3.5.5, p. 41) may reveal the site of bleeding or confirm the presence of blood in the stool (Table 22.1).

Piles and rectal carcinoma are very rare in children, and children with more than one episode without known cause should be seen in hospital. Colonoscopy is helpful. *Meckel's diverticulum* is an embryological remnant of the vitelline duct on the ileum and is present in 2% of the population, although in most it causes no symptoms. It often contains gastric mucosa which may ulcerate and bleed, causing rectal bleeding and anaemia. Radioactive technetium is selectively taken up by gastric mucosa and this provides the basis for an elegant diagnostic test.

22.2   Pathologies

22.2.1   The mouth

22.2.1.1   The teeth

There is considerable normal variation in the time of eruption of teeth, which may lead to unnecessary worry (Section 3.3). Preventative dental health is important for all children. Frequent sugary food should be avoided; we should not forget iatrogenic problems with medicines or vitamin drops. The bottle to suck while falling asleep or the dummy soaked in

Table 22.1 Causes of bleeding per rectum

Site	Condition	Clinical picture
Ileum	Intussusception	Colicky pain; redcurrant jelly stool; palpable mass
	Meckel's diverticulum	Intermittent abdominal pain and bleeding (red or melaena)
Colon	Dysentery (*Shigella, Salmonella*)	Acute mucoid diarrhoea and pain
	Ulcerative colitis	Chronic mucoid diarrhoea and pain
	Crohn's disease	Abdominal pain, diarrhoea and growth failure
	Intussusception	As above
Rectum	Polyp	Recurrent bleeding: no pain
	Prolapse	Prolapse visible
Anus	Fissure/constipation	On defaecation, much pain and little blood
	Sexual abuse	Dilated/sore anus

sweet fluid should be banned. Severe dental problems are more common in children with neurodevelopmental problems and in association with acid reflux.

Include the teeth in the examination of the mouth. It gives an opportunity for congratulation or health education.

Prevention of caries

↓**Plaque-forming organisms**
- Brushing and flossing

↓**Carbohydrates**
- Between meals
- At night

Adequate fluoride
- Supplemented drinking water
- Fluoride toothpaste

Regular dental supervision.

22.2.1.2 Cleft lip and palate

Cleft lip may be unilateral or bilateral (see Figure 8.6). It results from failure of fusion of the maxillary and frontonasal processes. In bilateral cases, the premaxilla (section of the upper lip just below the nose) is anteverted. There is always an associated nasal deformity (Section 8.4).

Cleft palate may occur alone or with cleft lip. It results from failure of fusion of the palatine processes and the nasal septum. Clefting causes nasal regurgitation of feeds and later 'cleft palate speech' because of nasal escape. Otitis media and sensorineural deafness are more common with clefts.

Special feeding techniques are often necessary. Submucous cleft palate, in which the muscle of the soft palate is cleft but the overlying mucosa is intact, is much less common. Always look for other congenital abnormalities.

Early referral to a multidisciplinary team (including orthodontists, plastic surgery, speech therapy) is needed. Most surgical repairs are done within the first 3 months.

22.2.1.3 Micrognathia and retrognathia

Some babies are born with a receding jaw, the mandible being either underdeveloped or displaced backward (Figure 22.4). In severe cases, the tongue (which is also abnormally far back) obstructs breathing from birth. In combination with cleft palate, this is known as *Pierre–Robin syndrome*. Problems with airway and feeding are most severe in early infancy. In most, mandibular growth and improved coordination lead to resolution.

22.2.1.4 Stomatitis

Risk factors for candidiasis

- Extreme prematurity
- Poor hygiene
- Broad-spectrum antibiotics
- Steroid inhalers
- Chronic illness
- Malnutrition
- Immunodeficiency
- HIV

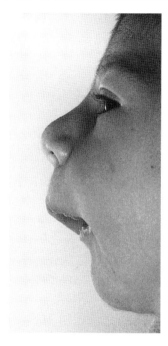

Figure 22.4 An infant with micrognathia and retrognathia.

Stomatitis due to *Candida albicans* (monilia: thrush) is common in infancy. It appears as tiny white flecks inside the cheeks, on the tongue and on the roof of the mouth (Figure 22.5). Milk curds are a little similar but are larger and can easily be detached with a spatula. *C.albicans* can be cultured from a swab, but treatment is often given on clinical grounds. *C.albicans* may also infect the skin of the napkin area (Figure 25.4).

 TREATMENT   Oral candidiasis

- Deal with risk factors
- Topical antifungal (e.g. nystatin, miconazole)
- Treat for a few days after apparent cure.

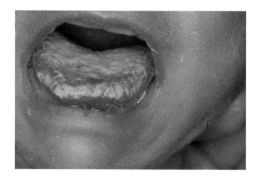

Figure 22.5 Oral thrush.

After infancy, stomatitis is usually due to a first infection with herpes simplex type 1 or coxsackie A virus (Section 15.3.3.2, p. 153). Treatment is mainly supportive, with maintenance of hydration, but oral acyclovir may be used for more severe cases if started within 3–4 days.

In *Stevens–Johnson syndrome*, severe mouth ulceration is associated with conjunctivitis, erythema multiforme and severe systemic illness.

22.2.2   Intestinal obstruction

 Bile-stained vomiting is obstruction until proven otherwise.

The causes of intestinal obstruction vary with age. In the younger child, fluid and electrolyte losses rapidly lead to dehydration and circulatory failure.

 Cardinal symptoms

- Vomiting ± bile
- Pain
- Abdominal distension
- Constipation.

 TREATMENT   Essential management

- Early diagnosis
- Correction of fluid and electrolyte losses
- Skilled surgery and anaesthesia.

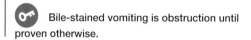 PRACTICE POINT

Gastrointestinal malformations present in the fetus or newborn. After infancy, inguinal hernia is the most common cause of bowel obstruction.

22.2.2.1   In the newborn

Fetal swallowing is essential for control of amniotic fluid volume. Obstruction high in the gastrointestinal tract leads to accumulation of fluid (polyhydramnios). No newborn infant with a history of polyhydramnios should be fed milk without ruling out oesophageal atresia (Figure 22.6).

 PRACTICE POINT   **Definitions**

- Atresia: passage not formed
- Stenosis: passage narrowed.

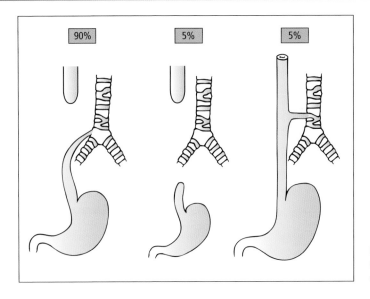

Figure 22.6 Three forms of oesophageal atresia ± tracheo-oesophageal fistula.

Oesophageal atresia is usually associated with *tracheo-oesophageal fistula*. Typically, there is polyhydramnios, and after birth the infant is 'bubbly' because saliva cannot be swallowed. Diagnosis must be made before milk is given as feeding will lead to choking, cyanosis and aspiration. This is a disastrous start in life for an infant who needs urgent surgery. If there is any suspicion of oesophageal atresia, a wide-bore nasogastric tube should be passed to demonstrate patency of the oesophagus. Early diagnosis and skilled surgery offer the best chance of cure. Other severe congenital abnormalities are present in about half the cases.

Atresias at lower levels cause vomiting and distension. In high obstruction, vomiting occurs early. Vomit contains bile if the obstruction is below the ampulla of Vater. *Duodenal atresia* and stenosis are particularly common in Down syndrome. *Rectal atresia* (imperforate anus) should not be missed on newborn examination. Infants with low, complete obstruction do not pass meconium, but those with high obstruction do.

Other congenital gut abnormalities

Hirschsprung disease is due to absence of the myenteric plexus in a segment of bowel, most commonly in the rectosigmoid region. Delayed passage of meconium is followed by constipation and distension. Rectal biopsy yields the diagnosis. Treatment is surgical.

In the embryo, the developing gut herniates from the abdominal cavity, returning with a twist so that the caecum ends up in the right iliac fossa. *Malrotation* occurs when this process is incomplete. It may result in obstruction from peritoneal bands compressing the intestine or *volvulus*. *Meconium ileus* is pathognomonic of CF (Section 20.8).

In *exomphalos*, the normal embryonic herniation development has become permanent. Bowel and other abdominal viscera protrude from the umbilicus, often enclosed in a membrane. *Gastroschisis* describes a serious congenital defect of the abdominal wall with herniation of peritoneal contents. Prior to surgical repair, a nasogastric tube is passed, fluid replacement is given and herniated intestine is wrapped in plastic.

22.2.2.2   Infancy and childhood

Intestinal obstruction at later ages may be caused by pyloric stenosis, intussusception, volvulus, strangulated inguinal hernia or other rare causes. Plain abdominal film may assist diagnosis (Figure 22.7).

Intussusception

 Intussusception

- Paroxysms of colicky pain
- Quiet and pale between attacks
- Cardinal features of obstruction (see box above)
- Redcurrant jelly stool (blood and mucus)
- Sausage-shaped mass (often right upper quadrant).

Intussusception occurs most commonly in infancy. Change in diet and intestinal flora or viral infection

OSCE station 22.1: Persistent diarrhoea

Task: You are to take a history from Kirsty's parent. Kirsty is 18 months of age and has had frequent loose stools for 3–4 months. The stools fill her nappy and overflow. She has no significant past medical history. The examiner will observe your history-taking, and at the end ask you what you think. Don't forget, take a full history but note:

Kirsty's history: key points

What are the stools like?	*Frequency, consistency and contents*	**Loose, pale and bulky stools.**
Any abnormal contents?	*Blood, mucus, parasites, undigested food, vegetables*	**Her stools are very offensive stools, but no blood.**
Associated symptoms?	*Vomiting, abdominal distension, mouth/ peri-anal disease*	**Stools do not flush away easily. Abdomen is always swollen.**
How is Kirsty?	*Is she her normal self otherwise? Is she energetic and playing and developing normally?*	**Always tired and moaning, and will not play for long.**
Dietary history?	*Is diet reasonable on quick assessment? Is there excessive fluid intake? What is fibre intake?*	**Diet is generally is normal and her appetite good.**
Growth?	*Parent-held record (red book): interpret growth chart*	**Weight and height have fallen from the 50–75th centiles. Weight now around 10th and height is 10–25th centile.**

Kirsty's history has important pointers to malabsorption and steatorrhoea. You cannot tell the cause from this history. It could be coeliac disease, CF or giardiasis. Many young children with persistent loose stools have toddler diarrhoea (Section 22.1.4) but would be growing normally.

OSCE station 22.2: Constipation

You are working in primary care as a junior trainee. Mrs McTaggart has brought her 7-year-old son James who has been soiling 3 times a week for a month. The GP, Dr Black, has diagnosed constipation, because James has been passing hard stools once a week for 4 months, and has significant faecal loading palpable in the abdomen. There is no history to suggest any other organic cause or any psychological upset. School are calling Mrs McTaggart in to help change James every time he soils, although when it occurs at home he usually sorts himself out without help. She has asked that you explain the diagnosis and agree a management plan with Mrs McTaggart. James is not present.

Introduction

Introduce yourself and your role, explain what you have been asked to do and confirm with Mrs McTaggart that she is happy with that. Brief clarifying questions will help to confirm key points in the history and set the scene for your explanation. checkIdeas, Concerns and Expectations (ICE).

Mrs McTaggart heard the GP mention constipation but is very sceptical. 'James' main problem is loose stools – how can that be constipation?' The GP mentioned laxatives, but 'Surely that will only make matters worse?' She will only be persuaded to agree to appropriate treatment if you give a clear and sympathetic explanation.

Explain the diagnosis

Explain that constipation is common, can build up gradually and does not need to have an obvious trigger. Explain the concept of overflow, and 'baggy' bowel (see Section 22.1.5). A diagram may be useful. Take time to address her concerns about the diagnosis and be clear why this is constipation. Ask if she has any other questions regarding diagnosis – *'Surely some investigations are needed?'* – explain that investigations are not necessary.

Management plan

- *General advice* – increased fibre, fluid and exercise. Deal with it in a low-key supportive way at school – talk to teacher about whether she could facilitate discreet access to a toilet, and James to take in clean pants and wipes.
- *Laxative disimpaction* – a stool softening osmotic agent (polyethylene glycol 3350 with electrolytes) to be taken in escalating daily doses until clearout (warn that soiling may get worse).
- *Laxative maintenance* – continue the stool softener regularly (1 paediatric sachet twice daily would be a reasonable dose), adjust up or down to achieve soft, formed daily stools. Continue for many months – if stopped too soon, the constipation will recur. A stimulant laxative (like senokot or picosulphate) is sometimes added after 2–3 weeks.
- *Sitting exercises and star chart* – James to get a star for sitting on the toilet and pushing for 3–5 minutes once or twice a day, 20 minutes after a meal. Another star for any stool passed in the toilet. Don't give stars for clean pants (could encourage with-holding). No withdrawal of stars or punishment for soiling – low-key, matter of fact approach.
- *Follow-up* – offer an early appointment in 2 weeks to review how things are going with the disimpaction.

Summarize and ask if any other questions

Summarize key points. Offer a leaflet. Ask if any questions.

What about side effects of the medication? Could he become addicted?

Reassure that the medication is safe, stays within the bowel and helps to hold water which softens, and is not addictive. The main problem is initial worsening of the soiling and/or diarrhoea, but this is a necessary stage of treatment. Also see OSCE station 4.1: 'Shock'.

SBAs

Q22.1 A 7-year-old boy presents with faecal soiling. This is on a background of constipation and he has painful episodes of passing hard stool as well. On examination he has a palpable faecal mass in the left iliac region. He has not on any current medication.

What is the most appropriate initial treatment?

a. Increase fibre in diet
b. Lactulose
c. Macrogol at a disimpaction dose
d. Phosphate enema
e. Star charts

Q22.2 A 4-year-old presents with gastroenteritis with mild (5%) dehydration. They are not in shock but are not tolerating oral fluids. They require treatment with intravenous (IV) fluids. Weight is 16 kg.

What is the appropriate hourly IV volume to prescribe if correcting the deficit over 24 hours?

a. 54 mls/h
b. 71 mls/h
c. 83 mls/h
d. 88 mls/h
e. 100 mls/h

For SBA answers, see page 368.

23

Urinary tract and genitalia

Chapter map

The commonest problems seen in primary and secondary care are urine infections, wetting problems and various concerns about the genitalia. Congenital problems are mainly picked up antenatally – posterior urethral valves are one of the most important. You should be able to recognize the classic paediatric presentations of acute nephritis and nephrotic syndrome and know an approach to presentations of haematuria and vaginal discharge. After a review of urinary tract development and urine examination, this chapter covers congenital abnormalities and then renal diseases, followed by urine infection and enuresis, and finishes with a section on genital problems.

Paediatrics Lecture Notes, Tenth Edition. Jonathan C. Darling and James Yong.
© 2022 John Wiley & Sons Ltd. Published 2022 by John Wiley & Sons Ltd.
Companion website: www.wiley.com/go/lecturenotes/paediatrics10e

23.5.6 Further investigation and management

PRACTICE POINT

The aim is to identify structural problems, scars and vesicoureteric reflux and to prevent or minimize future problems.

Younger children and those with atypical or recurrent infections (see Box) are investigated more thoroughly because of higher risk of problems. Older children with single, typical infections do not need investigation, but it is worth giving general advice about prevention. Recurrent infections that are a nuisance may be treated with prophylactic antibiotics.

Atypical and recurrent urine infections

Atypical UTI
- Seriously ill or sepsis
- Red flags (poor urine flow, abdominal mass, raised creatinine)
- Slow response to treatment (>48 h)
- Unusual organism (not *E. coli*)

Recurrent UTI
- ≥3 UTIs (or ≥2 if any upper tract infection)

  Prevention of UTIs

Regular water-drinking

Regular micturition

Avoid constipation

For girls:
- Check wiping from front to back (avoids gut flora reaching urethra)
- Avoid perineal irritation sometimes caused by bubble baths or strong soaps
- Regular washing and thorough drying of perineum
- Wear loose-fitting clothes (not tight trousers).

23.5.6.1 Renal ultrasound scan

- In children under six months or those with recurrent or atypical infections
- Identifies obstructive abnormalities and structural problems
- Assists diagnosis of acute pyelonephritis
- Discrepancies in renal size may indicate scarring.

23.5.6.2 Abdominal X-ray

Consider if there is suspicion of renal stones or spinal abnormalities.

23.5.6.3 Isotope scan (e.g. DMSA, MAG3)

- Perform in young children with atypical or recurrent infection
- Wait until 4-6 months after infection (otherwise hard to interpret)
- Inject i.v. radiolabelled isotope and visualize on scintigraphy
- Identifies renal scars and differential renal function
- Working renal tissue picks up the isotope and so a renal image is seen
- Scars show as blank areas
- Rate of excretion is seen as the kidney clears the isotope.

23.5.6.4 Micturating cystourethrogram (MCUG)

- Perform in infants <6 months with atypical or recurrent UTIs or when vesicoureteric reflux is suspected (e.g. other tests abnormal or family history)
- Catheterize bladder, fill with radio-opaque dye, watch on X-ray whilst child micturates
- Defines urethral abnormalities and vesicoureteric reflux (Table 23.4).

These are initial investigations. For young and ill children, the ultrasound should be done during the acute episode, otherwise within a few weeks. If any are abnormal, more investigations may be needed.

23.5.7 Vesicoureteric reflux

  Present in 1/4 children with urine infection

- Minor degrees unimportant
- When mild tends to resolve spontaneously
- Major reflux is a set-up for infection (Figure 23.5):
  - During micturition, urine refluxes up the ureter, filling and distending the calyces
  - At end of micturition urine falls back to form a stagnant pool.

Table 23.4 Investigation protocol for confirmed UTI

Age	Typical infection (not atypical or recurrent)	Atypical or recurrent infection
<6 months	USS	USS, DMSA, MCUG
6 months–3 years	None	USS, DMSA
Over 3 years	None	USS (+DMSA if recurrent)

Source: Based on the UK national guideline by the National Institute for Clinical Excellence (see CG54 at www.nice.org.uk) – last updated October 2018.

23.5.7.1 Management

- Prophylactic antibiotics to prevent infection
- Surgical correction is possible for severe or problematic reflux

    Follow-up important

- One-third have a recurrence of infection within a year
- Culture urine a few days after completing initial therapy
- Re-culture at least once in the next 3 months, even though the child is symptomless
- One of the causes of end-stage renal failure.

23.5.7.2 Prognosis

Infection of the renal parenchyma may cause permanent or progressive damage, leading to renal scarring, insufficiency and hypertension. Most children with UTI do not incur renal damage. Renal damage is most likely in those with associated obstruction of the urinary tract and in those who have severe infection and gross reflux early in life – under the age of 2.

23.6 Enuresis

Children learn to be dry by day at about 2 years and by night at about 3 years. By 4 years, 75% of children are dry by day and night. Most children who wet have 'intermittent' enuresis: it is rare to encounter children of school age who have never had a dry night.

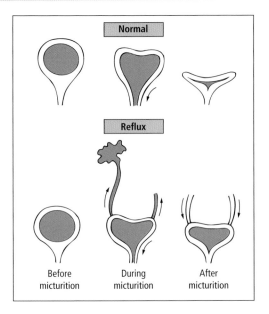

Figure 23.5 Vesicoureteric reflux (shown by micturating cystogram). At the end of micturition, a puddle of stagnant urine remains in the bladder.

Bedwetting (*nocturnal enuresis*) is a more common problem than daytime wetting (*diurnal enuresis*).

23.6.1 Nocturnal enuresis

Causes of nocturnal enuresis

- Lack of release of arginine vasopressin (ADH) during sleep with excess urine production
- Low functional bladder capacity
- Inability to wake to full bladder sensation
- Interference with learning (low IQ, delay, anxiety, unclear social approval/disapproval)
- Psychological distress: family dysfunction; bullying; abuse
- Medical conditions: urinary tract infection; constipation; diabetes mellitus; diabetes insipidus
- Inadvertent behavioural reinforcement (e.g. child comes into parents' bed when wet)
- Genetic factors (a positive family history is common).

Most enuretic children do not suffer from either a psychological illness or an organic illness.

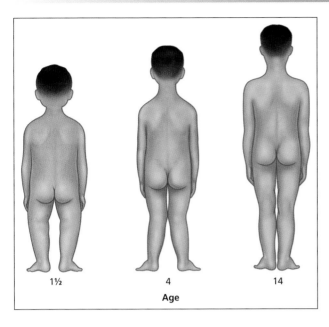

1½   4   14

Age

Figure 24.1 Normal variation of legs with age.

24.1.1 Flat feet

At birth, the feet look flat. A child's feet continue to look flat as a toddler. By the third year, the feet begin to appear to have a normal plantar arch.

24.1.2 Bow legs (genu varum)

Bow legs are most common from 0 to 2 years. The knees may be 5 cm apart when the feet are together: the toes point medially. Marked bowing may mean rickets (Section 13.4.2.4).

24.1.3 Knock knees (genu valgum)

This is most apparent at 3–4 years of age. When the knees are together, the medial tibial malleoli may be up to 5 cm apart. In obese children, the separation may be even greater but, by the age of 12, the legs should be straight. Separation of over 10 cm or unilateral knock knee requires an X-ray and, probably, a specialist opinion.

24.1.4 Intoeing

This is usually a normal variation and resolves by the age of 8 years.

24.1.5 Scoliosis

> **Causes of scoliosis**
> - Idiopathic (95%)
> - Vertebral anomalies, e.g. hemivertebrae
> - Muscle weakness, e.g. cerebral palsy.

Postural scoliosis is commonly seen in babies: it goes when the baby is suspended and has completely gone by the age of 2 years. Scoliosis is again common at adolescence, especially in girls. If it is postural, it disappears on bending forward. Structural scoliosis produces asymmetry on bending: a hump on flexion (Figure 24.2). Asymmetry of scapulae and shoulders may be more conspicuous than the spinal curve.

> **PRACTICE POINT**
>
> True (non-postural) scoliosis should be referred to orthopaedics promptly.

24.1.6 Talipes

Postural talipes is common at birth, resulting from the foetal foot position in utero. If the foot with talipes

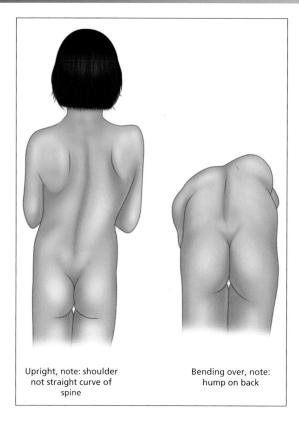

Upright, note: shoulder not straight curve of spine

Bending over, note: hump on back

Figure 24.2 Structural scoliosis becomes more obvious when she bends to touch her toes.

equinovarus (club foot) can be fully dorsiflexed and everted so that the little toe touches the outside of the leg without undue force, it is postural and will get better. Physiotherapy may be helpful. Structural talipes is harder to correct and early orthopaedic referral is needed. A series of leg casts over several months (Ponseti method) is usually successful, but some need surgery. The sooner treatment is begun the better the outcome. Talipes calcaneovalgus is usually easily corrected by simple exercises (Figure 24.3).

24.1.7 Developmental dysplasia of the hip (DDH)

DDH is also known as congenital dislocation of the hips. Acetabular dysplasia is important in causation.

Risk factors for DDH

- Breech
- Positive family history
- Girls > boys
- Neuromuscular or joint problem (e.g. spina bifida, talipes).

All babies should be examined in the neonatal period for DDH (OSCE station 24.1). Examination is repeated at infant health checks. If there is clinical suspicion or the infant is high risk, hip ultrasound is more reliable than clinical examination. X-ray is unreliable in the first months because of poor ossification.

- 1% of babies have some developmental dysplasia or hip instability
- 1 in 1000 have severe congenital dislocation
- early treatment with splinting in full abduction is successful in most
- late presentation with a limp has a poor prognosis, needing surgery and predisposing to early osteoarthritis.

 PRACTICE POINT

Screening tests for dislocated hips are not 100% sensitive (cases are missed) or 100% specific (the test may be abnormal in a normal infant).

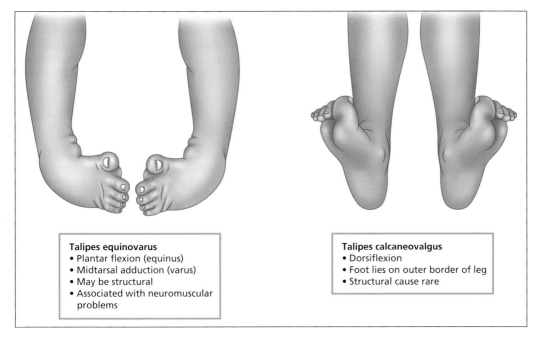

Talipes equinovarus
- Plantar flexion (equinus)
- Midtarsal adduction (varus)
- May be structural
- Associated with neuromuscular problems

Talipes calcaneovalgus
- Dorsiflexion
- Foot lies on outer border of leg
- Structural cause rare

Figure 24.3 Two forms of talipes.

24.1.8 Osteogenesis imperfecta

This is a group of rare genetic conditions due to mutations in the genes coding for collagen. They are characterized by brittle bones and lax ligaments. In the severe, lethal forms (dominant mutations or recessive inheritance), multiple fractures occur in utero. In less severe cases (usually dominant inheritance), children are prone to fractures, may have blue sclera and develop deafness in adult life (Figure 24.4).

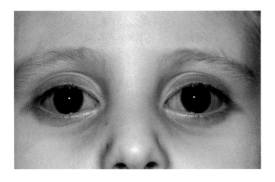

Figure 24.4 Osteogenesis imperfecta. The sclerae are blue in colour.

24.1.9 Skeletal dysplasia

These congenital dysplasias are rare. Many are genetically determined. *Achondroplasia* is the most common. It is due to an autosomal dominant gene. In 50% a new mutation occurs, both parents being normal. There is extreme short stature with disproportionate shortness of limbs, and a large skull vault. Intelligence is normal.

Some short-limbed dwarfism is incompatible with survival after birth (*thanatophoric*). Accurate diagnosis is important for genetic counselling.

24.2 Bone and joint infection

24.2.1 Osteomyelitis

Pyogenic infection of bone is more common in children than in adults, and in boys than in girls.

The usual site is the metaphysis of one of the long bones, particularly in the legs. *Staphylococcus aureus* is the most common pathogen.

Osteomyelitis

Symptoms
- Fever
- Variable pain, illness
- Pseudoparesis
- Local tenderness
- Redness, swelling

Investigations
- Blood count: neutrophilia
- C-reactive protein↑
- Blood culture
- Radioisotope scan
- X-ray.

- Early diagnosis is difficult: an infant may merely refuse to use the affected limb (pseudoparesis). X-ray is normal at first. After 2 weeks, bone rarefaction and periosteal new bone formation may be seen. Radioisotope bone scan is usually abnormal from the start.

Osteomyelitis demands intensive antibiotic treatment in hospital to try to prevent long-term effects on bone and joints. With early treatment, complete resolution occurs in most cases. If diagnosis is delayed, surgical drainage is more likely to be needed.

Flucloxacillin is the best antibiotic for most infections due to *S. aureus*. MRSA needs treatment with vancomycin.

24.2.2   Septic arthritis

Bacterial joint infection can occur at any age from the newborn. The most common cause is haematogenous spread of *S. aureus*. Symptoms and signs may be very like osteomyelitis. The affected joint is hot, swollen and immobile.

Early diagnosis is important for a good outcome. It is a difficult diagnosis in toddlers and infants especially when there is hip involvement. Septic arthritis should be managed with the orthopaedic surgeons. Joint aspiration usually provides a diagnosis. Joint lavage and drainage may be needed.

24.3   Arthritis and arthralgia

24.3.1   Transient synovitis of the hip (irritable hip)

This commonly is associated with viral infection. Unlike septic arthritis, the child is not usually ill, or

febrile. Pain is on walking and there are limited abduction and rotation. Infection screen and joint aspiration may be needed to exclude bacterial infection. Treatment is symptom relief, and improvement occurs in days.

24.3.2   Arthritis

 PRACTICE POINT   Arthritis

- Local pain
- Swelling
- Joint red and hot
- Limited movement.

Arthritis simply means inflammation in a joint, and there are many causes. If there is no history of joint swelling, arthritis is unlikely. Pain arising in the hip may be referred to as the knee. It is common in viral infections in children. Chronic arthropathy causes serious disability.

Causes of arthritis

Those that may result in permanent joint damage
- Juvenile idiopathic arthritis
- Acute septic arthritis
- Haemarthrosis (joint bleeding in coagulation disorders)

Those that usually resolve completely
- Reactive arthritis: viral infections
  - Rubella
  - Immunization
  - Mumps
- Henoch–Schönlein syndrome
- Generalized allergic reactions
- Rheumatic fever.

24.3.2.1   Juvenile idiopathic arthritis (JIA, juvenile chronic arthritis)

JIA classification

- Systemic-onset (previously known as Still's)
- Polyarticular
- Pauciarticular
- Psoriatic
- Enthesitis-related

JIA is defined as a chronic arthritis before the age of 16 years, lasting at least 6 weeks, after exclusion of other primary diseases. Children do not always easily fit into one of the classifications.

Systemic disease (Still's)
- Preschool children
- Generally unwell
- Swinging, high fever
- Splenomegaly
- Lymphadenopathy
- Erythematous (salmon pink) rash
- High CRP
- Polymorph leucocytosis
- Rheumatoid/antinuclear factors negative

Polyarticular JIA
- Any age
- Over four joints
- Symmetrical
- Hands, wrists, knees, ankles
- No systemic inflammation

Pauciarticular JIA
- Young children
- Up to four joints
- Knees, ankles, elbows
- Muscle wasting
- Antinuclear antibody positive
- Risk of uveitis.

Rarely children develop juvenile rheumatoid arthritis with a typical pattern of hand and even cervical spine involvement and with positive rheumatoid factor (RF+). Enthesitis means inflammation at the site of tendon insertion. In enthesitis, large joint arthritis and iritis also occur, mostly in older boys who are HLA type B27. Psoriatic arthritis may start well before the rash – suspect it if nail-pitting, or a first degree relative with the condition.

 TREATMENT   Management of JIA

- Multidisciplinary team is key!
- Physiotherapy
- Non-steroidal anti-inflammatory drugs
- Local/systemic steroids
- Methotrexate
- Anti-cytokine antibodies ('biologics').

Prognosis depends on type (worse with polyarthritis, RF+) but is improving with biologic agents. Fifty per cent of children attain remission within 5 years, but for some, the disease is still progressive and crippling. Iridocyclitis is an important complication.

24.3.3   Joint hypermobility syndrome

Children with very mobile joints may suffer pain after exercise, or after prolonged sitting. Symptoms are often worse around the adolescent growth spurt. When mild, reassurance and general advice about posture and pacing activity is all that is necessary. More severe cases need evaluation for collagen disease and may benefit from physiotherapy.

24.3.4   Other collagen diseases

Systemic lupus erythematosus (SLE), polyarteritis nodosa, dermatomyositis and the other collagen disorders are rare in children. SLE tends to occur in adolescent girls, particularly in black races. It tends to present as a multisystem disorder and responds well to treatment with corticosteroids.

24.3.5   Henoch–Schönlein purpura (anaphylactoid purpura)

HSP

- Most common in children aged 2–10 years
- Vasculitic process
- Involves the following four organ systems:
  - Skin – pathognomonic purpuric rash
  - Joints
  - Gut
  - Kidneys.

24.3.5.1   Skin

The rash is distributed over the extensor surfaces of the limbs, particularly the ankles and the buttocks (Figure 24.5). It begins as a maculopapular, red rash, which gradually becomes purpuric (resulting from the vasculitis, the platelet count is normal). Swelling of the face, hands and feet is common.

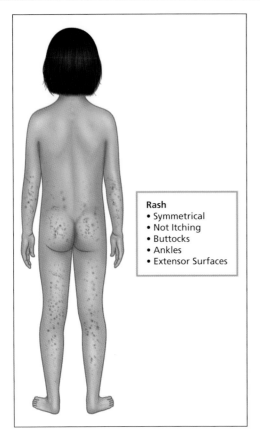

Rash
- Symmetrical
- Not Itching
- Buttocks
- Ankles
- Extensor Surfaces

Figure 24.5 Henoch–Schönlein purpura.

24.3.5.2 Joints

Pain (arthralgia) of medium-sized joints is common and may progress to an obvious arthritis with red, swollen, tender joints.

24.3.5.3 Alimentary system

Colicky abdominal pain occurs and may be severe enough to mimic an acute abdominal emergency. Vomiting and diarrhoea are common, haematemesis and melaena less common. Intussusception may occur (Section 22.2.2.2, p. 252). Perforation is very rare.

24.3.5.4 Kidneys

Renal injury is caused by deposition of IgA immune complexes. Haematuria is common but, when accompanied by persisting proteinuria, is of concern. With more severe involvement, the glomerulonephritis causes an acute nephritic syndrome or nephrotic syndrome. Acute or chronic renal failure may occur in

a small minority. The renal complications are responsible for the main morbidity and mortality of Henoch–Schönlein syndrome.

 PRACTICE POINT

In HSP, dipstick urine for blood and protein (parents are asked to do this at home for a few weeks), and measure BP.

HSP usually resolves after 1–3 weeks. The cause is unknown, and treatment is symptomatic. Recurrence may occur for several months after onset. Steroids may be helpful for severe gastrointestinal and renal involvement.

24.3.6 Rheumatic fever

Rheumatic fever is still an important cause of acquired heart disease in children throughout the world, but in Europe, it has become rare. It results from a sensitivity reaction to a group A β-haemolytic streptococcal infection usually after acute tonsillitis (Figure 24.6). Treatment includes antibiotics, anti-inflammatory agents and long-term penicillin prophylaxis against recurrence.

Rheumatic fever
- Transient arthritis
- Pancarditis
- Cardiac valve damage
- Rash (erythema marginatum)
- Erythema nodosum
- Chorea
- High ASO titre.

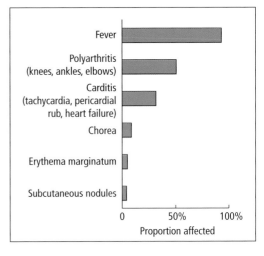

Figure 24.6 Rheumatic fever signs.

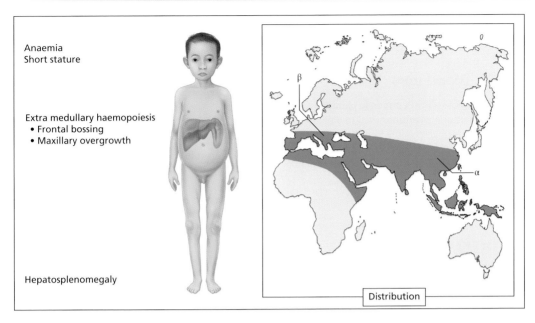

Anaemia
Short stature

Extra medullary haemopoiesis
• Frontal bossing
• Maxillary overgrowth

Hepatosplenomegaly

Distribution

Figure 26.2 Thalassaemia major.

ders. HbS is present in place of HbA. At low oxygen tensions, the cell becomes crescent- or sickle-shaped and is likely to haemolyse. Heterozygotes have about 30% HbS, may show sickling, but are usually well. Homozygotes develop recurrent episodes of haemolysis (crises) from infancy. Thromboses in mesenteric, intracranial or bone vessels produce severe pain (painful crisis), simulating acute abdominal emergencies, meningitis or arthritis. Hydroxycarbamide (which increases HbF and improves blood flow) is used if there are frequent painful episodes.

Sickle cell disease

Anaemia
Acute crises
• Painful, vaso-occlusive
• Haemolytic
• Sequestration
• Aplastic (post-parvovirus)
Infection (e.g. pneumococcus)
Dactylitis (hand–foot syndrome).

Although prognosis has improved with screening and improved management, death in late childhood or early adult life from infections, cardiac failure or thrombotic episodes may still occur. The outlook is

 TREATMENT

Painful crises need:
• Analgesia
• Oxygen
• Hydration
• Warmth.

better if general health and nutrition are good. DNA probes are available for prenatal diagnosis and carrier detection. There is universal newborn screening in the UK.

 RESOURCE POINTER

See **www.nice.org.uk** and search 'sickle cell' or CG143 for UK guidance.

26.2.2.4   Extracellular abnormalities

Antibodies causing destruction of the red cell are usually associated with a positive Coombs' test. The only common example in childhood is haemolytic disease of the newborn (Section 9.4.2.1, p. 92). Rarer causes include severe poisoning or infection, malignancy and systemic lupus erythematosus.

26.2.3 Blood loss

Hidden blood loss is not common in childhood: peptic ulcers, piles and gastrointestinal malignancy are rare. Gastrointestinal bleeding from a Meckel's diverticulum or reflux oesophagitis is more likely to present with overt bleeding than unexplained anaemia.

26.3 Coagulation disorders

26.3.1 Haemophilia (Table 26.2)

Haemophilia A is over five times more common than B. Both are only seen in boys. Severity is related to the degree of deficiency of the relevant factor. In haemophilia A, symptoms occur with less than 10% of normal clotting activity. Severe disease occurs with <1%. Prolonged partial thromboplastin time leads to a specific assay of the relevant coagulation factor (Prothrombin time is normal.)

26.3.1.1 Presentation

- Excessive bruising as the boy learns to crawl and walk during the second year.
- Prolonged bleeding following circumcision, blood sampling or tooth eruption.

26.3.1.2 Treatment

Bleeding episodes are treated and prevented by intravenous injection of factor concentrate; most families manage their own injections. Traumatic contact sports are forbidden, but an active, enjoyable life is encouraged. Haemarthroses (bleeding into a joint), especially of the ankle and knees, can lead to permanent joint damage. Haemorrhage after dental extraction and other surgical procedures can be avoided by factor replacement.

Table 26.2 Haemophilia

Haemophilia	Deficient factor	Inheritance
A	VIII	X-linked recessive
B (Christmas disease)	IX	X-linked recessive

🔑 Before 1985, some factor VIII was contaminated with HIV. Many haemophiliacs died of AIDS. Factors VIII and IX are now manufactured with recombinant genetic technologies, rather than from blood.

Haemophilia usually becomes less severe as an adult. Regional haemophilia centres provide expert care and provide a service for prenatal diagnosis and the identification of female carriers.

Von Willebrand syndrome affects both boys and girls, with autosomal dominant inheritance. Though there is a combination of factor VIII deficiency and platelet dysfunction, the degree of bleeding disorder is usually mild.

26.3.2 Thrombocytopenia

The most common thrombocytopenic purpura of childhood is *idiopathic thrombocytopenic purpura* (ITP) (Table 26.3). The onset is acute, often occurring 1–3 weeks after an upper respiratory tract infection. A widespread petechial rash appears, developing into small purpuric spots (Figure 26.3). There may be bleeding from the nose or into the mucous membranes. Serious internal or intracranial bleeds are rare.

Table 26.3 Main causes of purpura in children

Platelet count low (thrombocytopenia)	Platelet count normal
Idiopathic thrombocytopenic purpura	Septicaemia (particularly meningococcal)
Leukaemia (Chapter 27)	Henoch–Schönlein purpura (Chapter 24)
Disseminated intravascular coagulation	Common viral infections
Toxic effect of drugs	

ITP

Hb normal
WBC normal
Platelets low (<30 × 10⁹/L)
Marrow shows ↑ immature megakaryocytes.

Generally, the outcome is good. Seventy-five per cent of children make a complete recovery within a month. Transfusions of platelets and blood are rarely needed. In severe cases with persistent bleeding, corticosteroids

---

Causes of hypoglycaemia

Hormonal
- Excess insulin
- Lack of cortisol (e.g. congenital adrenal hyperplasia).

Metabolic
- Ketotic hypoglycaemia
- Liver disease
- Glycogen storage disorders
- Galactosaemia
- Other inborn errors of metabolism.

28.3 Thyroid disease

Normal thyroid function is necessary for healthy physical and mental growth.

28.3.1 Congenital hypothyroidism

This is usually due to the absence of the thyroid gland. Occasionally, a small or ectopic thyroid is present, or metabolic problems in the gland prevent production of thyroid hormone. Neonatal screening at the end of the first week of life measures thyroid-stimulating hormone (TSH), which is raised. Very rarely hypothyroidism is due to panhypopituitarism and TSH levels are normal or low.

This successful screening programme allows early instigation of lifelong hormone replacement therapy with oral thyroxine. The untreated child with very short stature, coarse features, scanty hair, an umbilical hernia and severe learning problems is now a feature of history.

28.3.2 Juvenile hypothyroidism

Later thyroid failure is more common in children with diabetes and in those with Down or Turner syndromes. The cardinal feature is a fall-off in physical growth (Section 14.1.2). Symptoms are very similar to those seen in the adult, with school failure and learning problems. Juvenile hypothyroidism is normally due to autoimmune disease, and autoantibodies are present. Rarely, it is of pituitary origin.

Children with Down syndrome may be screened annually for hypothyroidism and coeliac disease as both are more common and difficult to recognize.

28.3.3 Hyperthyroidism and goitre

A transient form of this occurs in newborn infants who receive IgG transplacentally from a mother who has a history of *Graves' disease* (autoimmune hyperthyroidism often associated with exophthalmos).

Goitre may occur in adolescent girls who are euthyroid. Classical Graves' disease is unusual in children.

28.4 The adrenal glands

Disorders of the adrenal gland are uncommon in children. The least rare is congenital adrenal hyperplasia. *Addison disease* (hypoadrenalism), presenting later in life with growth failure and hyperpigmentation, is very rare. Cushing syndrome, the result of excess corticosteroid activity, is almost always the result of therapeutic use of steroids. Rarely, adrenal cortical tumours secrete androgens or oestrogens, with consequent early appearance of secondary sexual characteristics (adrenarche).

28.4.1 Congenital adrenal hyperplasia

This results from a metabolic block in the synthesis of hydrocortisone. The 21-hydroxylase enzyme is absent in children who are homozygous for an autosomal recessive gene mutation. There are two consequences:

- Absence of sufficient circulating corticosteroids and mineralocorticoids
- ↑ pituitary ACTH → adrenal cortical hypertrophy → ↑ androgens.

Clinical features depend on the child's sex. Girls are virilized with abnormal genitalia, enlarged clitoris and labia fusion, which may prevent accurate determination of sex at birth. Boys have normal genitalia. The majority of children with this condition lack mineralocorticoids and present in the first weeks because of salt loss. Typically, they have a history of vomiting and are markedly dehydrated. Some are severely ill, and the condition is lethal if not recognized and treated.

Diagnosis is made by finding elevated levels of cortisone precursors (17-hydroxyprogesterone) and, in salt losers, a low serum sodium and an elevated potassium. Treatment is lifelong hormone replacement therapy. The dose must be increased at times of illness and stress. Girls may require genital plastic surgery.

PRACTICE POINT

If a newborn infant is not clearly male or female, do not assign the sex until clarified through further investigation. This is awkward, but better than discovering that a boy is in fact a girl.

28.4.2 Cushing syndrome

Features of Cushing syndrome
- Round, fat face
- Obesity
- Poor growth
- Hypertension
- Osteoporosis.

The effects of excess glucocorticoid are almost always due to steroid treatment (Figure 28.2). Long-term steroid therapy should only be used when it is essential. *Cushing disease* (primary excess steroid secretion by the child's own adrenals) and other causes of endogenous excess glucocorticoids are rare. The combination of obesity and reduced height/growth should raise suspicion.

 PRACTICE POINT

Short obese children are more likely to have an endocrine problem than those who are tall or of average height.

28.5 Growth hormone deficiency

Deficiency of growth hormone (GH) is an uncommon, but important, cause of growth failure. It may be isolated or associated with deficiency of other pituitary hormones. It is sometimes secondary to an intracranial lesion.

Lack of response to stimulation of GH secretion is diagnostic. In the GH stimulation test, clonidine or glucagon is given and blood samples are taken over a few hours. Often, thyroid and pituitary function tests are done at the same time.

Genetically engineered human GH is given by injection, under expert supervision and close monitoring. GH is sometimes used to treat short children without deficiency (e.g. Turner syndrome, achondroplasia).

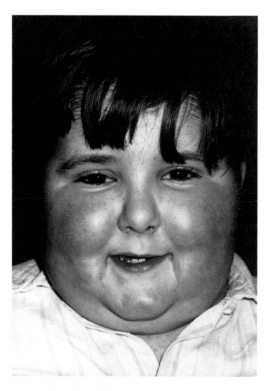

Figure 28.2 Steroid therapy has led to obesity, a round face and hirsuteness.

28.6 Diabetes insipidus

In this rare condition, antidiuretic hormone (ADH) is not produced or does not work. There is marked thirst and the passage of large volumes of dilute urine of low osmolality. There is constant danger of serious water depletion, especially in hot weather.

 Central diabetes insipidus

Hypothalamus not producing ADH.

 Nephrogenic diabetes insipidus

Renal tubule not responding to ADH.

Part 4

After paediatrics

This chapter takes you beyond your paediatric placement. You will need to prepare for exams, and we give you tips and pointers for paediatric examinations in Chapter 29.

It won't be long before you are prescribing, including for children. It is worth keeping this in mind throughout your time in paediatrics. Prescribing for children has unique risks, and we highlight these in Chapter 30.

Chapter 31 gives some careers advice – we hope of interest to many readers!

The final chapter provides self-test questions (with answers and explanations) which we hope will be a useful way to review what you have learnt.

Preparing for clinical examinations in paediatrics and child health

Chapter map

Although we hope that you are learning about paediatrics and child health because it is an interesting and enjoyable subject, we know that you want to pass clinical examinations in the subject. The purpose of this chapter is to give you specific help with how to prepare for such examinations. There are currently many modes of assessment in under-graduate paediatric examinations, but they divide into written and clinical examinations.

29.1 Clinical examinations

Traditionally, these consisted of a long case and several short cases, but such formats have been criticized for lacking objectivity and reproducibility, and for inadequate sampling of students' skills. They are very close to what you will do in real practice, and encourage a thoughtful, integrative and patient-centred approach to clinical skills. In an Objective Structured Clinical Examination (OSCE) (see below), you are asked to demonstrate a variety of clinical skills, but it is harder for examiners to make sure that you can put a whole series of skills together and make sense of the outcome. Some medical schools use an exam format that is part way between long and short cases, where you might be partly observed taking a history or examining a patient (or both) in a shortened time frame and then be asked questions about diagnosis and management.

29.1.1 Objective Structured Clinical Examinations (OSCEs)

These have become the most widely used method of assessing clinical skills, because they allow all students to be assessed performing the same tasks in the same

Paediatrics Lecture Notes, Tenth Edition. Jonathan C. Darling and James Yong.
© 2022 John Wiley & Sons Ltd. Published 2022 by John Wiley & Sons Ltd.
Companion website: www.wiley.com/go/lecturenotes/paediatrics10e

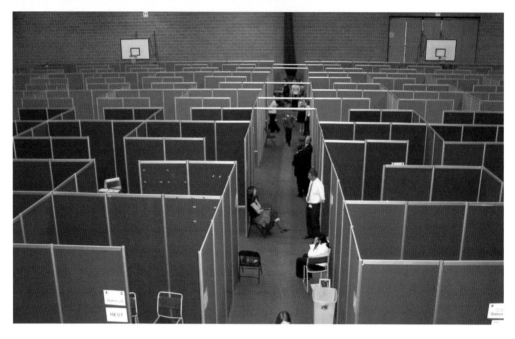

Figure 29.1 An OSCE examination with multiple circuits all running simultaneously.

or similar clinical situations, with objective marking criteria and wide sampling of skills. In an OSCE, candidates rotate around stations, with a preset time of between 5 and 20 min allowed for each (Figure 29.1). Stations will range over a variety of clinical skills.

The principle is simple. The examiners first determine what is required of the candidate. A standardized question is given to the candidate (e.g. please examine this 4-year-old boy's cardiovascular system), and the candidate is observed by the examiner, who grades essential elements as they are performed. Further marks are given for general approach, rapport with the child and their parent (or proxy parent), and interpretation of the findings.

A badly written OSCE station will allow you to accumulate marks by a haphazard approach, where you do everything you can possibly think of in a thoughtless and random order. Such stations are now rare. To gain high marks in a good OSCE station, you need to demonstrate a logical approach, good communication and examination skills, and then show that you are able to synthesize and make sense of the clinical information.

 OSCE TIP   Examples of clinical skills tested in OSCE stations

Communication (sometimes with a proxy parent)
- History-taking
- History presentation and discussion
- Counselling and explaining

Physical examination (with a patient, manikin or video)
- Systems examination, e.g. CVS, respiratory, abdomen, joints, neurology (part), gait, squint, ENT (manikin), newborn hips (manikin)
- Developmental assessment
- Assessment of peak flow or use of asthma devices

Practical and emergency skills
- Practical tasks without a patient (dipstick testing of urine)
- Prescribing
- Resuscitation (manikin).

each patient or clinical scenario. A number of *stems* will follow, describing patients who present with the problem given in the theme. Question banks will often contain stems that correspond to each option in the option list, although when the question is featured in an exam, only a small number of the stems may be presented. The description given in the stem should be such that if you have gained reasonable clinical experience of that problem, you will be able to state the correct answer *without looking at the option list*.

EMQ tips

1. Read the theme, lead-in and first stem, but not the option list initially.
2. Imagine yourself in the clinical situation given, for example seeing a child on the ward, in out-patients or in A&E, and try and decide what the most likely answer would be in that setting.
3. Now look at the option list and see if your answer features there.
4. Check the other options to see if any others would be a reasonable alternative answer and if so decide which of these is the most likely.
5. If you cannot come up with the answer without looking at the option list, then work through them and see if you can work out the correct option by a process of exclusion.
6. You may notice that several of the options could not apply.

29.2.3 Single Best Answer questions

These consist of a stem (such as a clinical scenario), a lead-in question, followed by a series of options (typically one correct and four distractors). Note that the incorrect options may not be entirely wrong, but one will be 'most correct' e.g. the most likely diagnosis. These are broadly similar to Extended Matching Questions above, but with a single scenario per option set. The same approach as that recommended for EMQs above applies. We have included Single Best Answer questions for self-testing at the end of most chapters.

29.2.4 Multiple-choice questions

This has been a common question format for years, and there are many sources of example questions.

MCQs test your factual knowledge over a broad area in a short space of time. A number of tips can allow you to benefit from flaws in question writing. However, increasingly, such flaws are recognized by question reviewers and will be edited out before the question gets to you. Then you have to depend on your factual knowledge, which is how it should be. Don't forget to read questions carefully and avoid jumping to conclusions.

MCQ tips

- Responses that state the something 'never' occurs or 'always' occurs are unlikely to be correct.
- Responses that don't follow grammatically from the stem are more likely to be incorrect.
- Options that are significantly longer than the rest are more likely to be correct.
- Options that repeat words from the stem are more likely to be correct.

29.2.5 Clinical image questions

These may be questions based on pictures projected as slides or printed in a question book. The questions may be in short answer format or you may be asked to select the best option from many, particularly for computer-marked exams. Where there are follow-on questions, there may well be clues to the answers of previous questions. Therefore, it is worth reading the whole question set before committing yourself on paper. This sort of question type has often been a feature of paediatric OSCE examinations where you may be presented with a piece of equipment, a picture of a patient or an X-ray and asked to answer questions about it. Most such questions can be converted into a written paper, computer-marked format.

Clinical image tips

- Being regularly around clinical areas will help you in your preparation for such papers.
- Make sure you are familiar with all common pieces of equipment and other items used in the care of children that you might see on the wards or in out-patients (Figure 29.2).
- Review pictures in this book, and paediatric atlases, focusing particularly on common and important problems that manifest in a way that can be photographed.

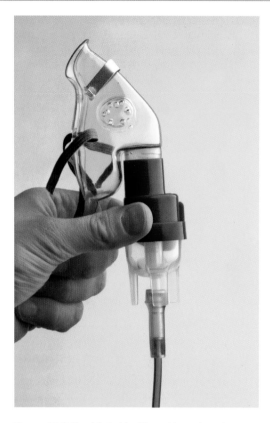

Figure 29.2 Be able to identify and know how to use commonly used equipment in paediatrics, for example this is a nebulizer mask.

29.2.6 Short answer questions and data interpretation

In this question format, you may be presented with some data (e.g. a set of results, or a pedigree), or a clinical image with some background clinical information. You are then asked a series of questions to which there are succinct answers, for example 'What is the most likely diagnosis?', or 'Suggest the three most appropriate next investigations'. Again, take time to read the whole question. If you think you know the answers, be as precise as you can (e.g. '*left upper lobe* pneumonia', not just 'pneumonia').

29.2.7 Essays

These are an unusual feature of undergraduate examination in paediatrics, because marking is less objective and more time-consuming. Some courses use 'modified-essay' questions, for example where you

Short answer tips

1. If three options are asked for, give exactly three, and never more.
2. Keep your answers precise and clear.
3. Imagine yourself dealing with the real clinical problem in out-patients or A&E.
4. Make a list of the various categories that can cause disease (sometimes called a 'surgical or aetiological sieve' – see Section 4.2). Go through each category and decide whether it could contain an explanation to the problem.
5. Look carefully at *all* the clinical information you have (including later questions).
6. Look for a single diagnosis that will explain all the features.

are asked to write short notes on a topic in 15 min. These are good for testing your approach to complex but important clinical situations, for example 'Describe key aspects of the management of a child with diabetic ketoacidosis'. They can also be used to test areas that do not lend themselves to testing in computer-marked formats, for example 'Describe the potential ill-effects of admitting a 3-year-old child to hospital for a 3-day course of intravenous antibiotics for a urine infection, and how these may be minimized'. Those marking your responses are likely to have a pre-prepared scheme with key points for which they will award marks. It is well worth jotting down as many key points as you can before you start formally answering the question. Vague answers that keep repeating the same points will not do well.

 # Summary

Paediatrics is a clinical subject, and to do well in examinations, you need to do plenty of clinical practice. You need a basic grounding of factual knowledge, which you will find in a textbook such as this one, but you need to take every opportunity to put that knowledge into practice in real clinical situations. Once you have become proficient in all the basic paediatric clinical skills through frequent practice, you are likely to improve your examination outcomes further through attention to technique, and practice that is specifically targeted at the exam format used in your undergraduate course.

Answer to EMQ example earlier in this chapter: 1D, 2A, 3B

D. Mouth-to-mouth ventilation

E. Oral airway

F. Tracheal intubation and ventilation

In each of the following cases, select the most appropriate airway procedure. Assume all the equipment needed for each procedure is to hand:

7. A newborn infant needs resuscitation. He is given bag and mask ventilation, but his pulse remains <100 bpm, he is pale and not breathing.

8. A 2-year-old is admitted in status epilepticus. Fits are terminated with intravenous lorazepam. As the fits stop, the child makes some croaking sounds, his chest continues to move, but he is becoming blue.

9. On her third birthday, a child suddenly becomes distressed at her party, while playing a game with sweets. She runs to her mother looking terrified and is clearly not breathing.

10. A 10-year-old boy is knocked off his bike at traffic lights. You see him go through the air and land on the road. When you get there, he is not breathing.

Foetal medicine (Chapter 7)

EMQ 7.1 Foetal diagnoses

A. Down syndrome

B. Hydrops fetalis

C. Intrauterine growth restriction (IUGR)

D. Macrosomia (growth greater than 95th centile)

E. Tracheo-oesophageal fistula

F. Urethral valves

For each of the following, choose which foetal condition is most likely:

11. A woman has pregnancy-induced hypertension with proteinuria and oedema (pre-eclampsia). There is placental insufficiency, and ultrasound shows oligohydramnios (reduced amniotic liquor).

12. Foetal ultrasound shows reduced liquor and dilated urinary tract with a full bladder. The baby needs to be delivered in a centre which can provide surgery.

13. A woman is found to have polyhydramnios (excess liquor). Foetal growth is normal. At birth, the infant is in good condition, but is bubbly and mucousy and needs oral suction twice.

14. A woman of 37 years is pregnant. Foetal ultrasound at 17 weeks shows thickening of the back of the neck (nuchal fold). The foetus appears otherwise normal.

15. A 28-year-old woman has gestational diabetes. Her diabetic control is less good in the third trimester and her fundal height (size of uterus) is large for dates.

16. In her third pregnancy, a woman is found to have anti-Rhesus D antibodies in her blood. Foetal ultrasound shows ascites. Arrangements are made for foetal blood transfusion because the foetus has become anaemic.

Birth and the newborn infant (Chapter 8)

EMQ 8.1 Examination of the newborn

A. Cephalhaematoma

B. Erythema toxicum

C. Stork mark

D. Strawberry naevus

E. Subaponeurotic haemorrhage

F. Traumatic cyanosis

For each of the following, choose the most likely diagnosis:

17. At 2 days of age, a baby has a widespread red rash, which has appeared rapidly. Each spot has a yellow centre. Some of the spots present this morning are no longer visible.

18. A baby's mother is concerned about a red mark between her daughter's eyebrows. It is more visible when the baby cries and goes onto the upper eyelids.

19. A newborn baby has swelling over the left side of his head. He appears generally well.

20. A 6-week-old infant had no birthmarks at birth. Mother has now noticed a bright red, pea-sized lump over the upper arm. It is getting bigger.

21. After ventouse vacuum delivery, this infant is found to be unwell at 8 h. She is pale, and quiet, with a raised respiratory rate. Her head feels boggy all over.

EMQ 8.2 Management of neonatal problems

A. Admit the baby to the neonatal unit

B. Reassure and arrange community or outpatient follow-up

C. Reassure but arrange to review the infant next day

D. Reassure the mother, no action is needed

E. Refer to the surgeon

For each of the following, choose the most appropriate management:

22. A 12-h-old baby is noted to have a full fontanelle when he cries. Otherwise, he is well and the fontanelle feels normal when he is quiet.

23. A newborn baby boy has an abnormal foreskin, which is gathered around the dorsal surface of the glans.

24. A 4-h-old girl has a respiratory rate of 75/min and has a quiet expiratory grunt. Examination otherwise is entirely normal.

25. A 1-day-old girl has numerous small white spots over her nose.

26. At the routine examination, you notice that a baby's head circumference is 1 cm over the 99.8th centile.

Disorders of the newborn (Chapter 9)

EMQ 9.1 Definitions used in neonatal medicine

A. Appropriate weight for gestational age

B. Large for gestational age

C. Low birthweight

D. Postmature

E. Preterm

F. Small for gestational age

G. Term

H. Very low birthweight

Classify each of the following using one or more of the definitions above. You will need to use the growth chart (Chapter 9, Figure 9.1). **More than one of the terms above may apply to each infant.**

27. An infant born at 34 weeks gestation with a weight of 1.6 kg.

28. An infant born at 41 weeks gestation with a weight of 3.7 kg.

29. An infant born at 29 weeks gestation with a weight of 1.2 kg.

EMQ 9.2 Respiratory problems in the newborn

A. Congenital diaphragmatic hernia

B. Congenital heart malformation

C. Group B streptococcal pneumonia

D. Meconium aspiration syndrome

E. Pneumothorax

F. Respiratory distress syndrome

G. Transient tachypnoea of the newborn

For each of the following, choose the most likely diagnosis:

30. Peter is 1.9 kg at 31 weeks gestation. He is tachypnoeic at 2 h of age, needing 40% oxygen to maintain good oxygen saturation.

31. Catherine was born at term, 28 h after rupture of membranes. She appeared well, but now at 6 h the midwife notes a raised respiratory rate, and Catherine is not interested in feeding.

32. Lawrence was delivered by elective caesarean section at 39 weeks. He was tachypnoeic 20 min after delivery, but on review, 25 min later he has less respiratory distress.

33. Simon is born at term. He has respiratory distress with cyanosis from birth. Air entry is difficult to hear on the left side and his abdomen is very flat. He becomes pink with oxygen.

EMQ 9.3 Neonatal problems

A. Preterm infant, appropriate for gestational age

B. Small for gestational age infant born at term

C. Term infant after intrapartum asphyxia

D. Term infant of a mother with diabetes

E. Term infant who is small for gestational age

Which infant or infants are most likely to have the following problems (more than one option may be appropriate)?

34. At 7 h, this infant is increasingly jittery. She is pale, sweaty and floppy, and will not feed.

35. At 6 h, this infant begins to have fits and appears floppy and unresponsive.

36. This infant's mother was unwell in the first trimester. At term after birth, he is noted to have cataracts and microcephaly.

37. This infant has a birthweight of 1.3 kg, and after 7 days of intensive care for respiratory distress syndrome, the baby deteriorates. A loud systolic murmur is heard and her pulses are bounding.

EMQ 9.4 Management of neonatal jaundice

A. Double phototherapy and prepare for exchange transfusion
B. Investigate for biliary atresia
C. Phototherapy and repeat bilirubin
D. Reassure parents and observe

For each infant, choose the most appropriate management:

38. James is 3 days old and has visible jaundice; he appears well. His bilirubin level is above the line for phototherapy on the chart.

39. Billy is 12 days old, appears healthy and is breast-feeding well. He is still jaundiced. His stools are normal.

40. At 4 h, Sally is jaundiced. Her mother had raised anti-D antibody levels. Sally's haemoglobin is 8 g/dL, and her bilirubin is high.

41. Marie is 18 days old, and she is still jaundiced. She appears well, taking regular formula feeds. Her stools are pale off-white.

Child development and how to assess it (Chapter 10)

EMQ 10.1 Types of developmental delay

A. Normal
B. Gross motor delay
C. Fine motor delay
D. Language delay
E. Gross motor and fine motor delay
F. Gross motor and language delay
G. Fine motor and language delay
H. Global delay

For each child, select the most appropriate description.

42. A 20-month-old boy is cruising around furniture but not yet taking any steps. He can pull to stand and has been sitting on his own since about age 12 months. He has about 20 clear words and some two-word sentences. He understands simple commands and his parents have no concerns about his hearing. He can scribble with a crayon, but cannot copy a line. He can build a tower of four cubes.

43. A 4-year-old walked at age 19 months and falls often when he tries to run. He cannot kick a ball, ride a trike or jump. He can copy a line, but not a circle or a cross. He cannot copy a three-brick 'gate' or six-brick 'steps', but can copy a four-brick 'train'. He knows about 300 words and speaks in sentences of 5–10 words.

44. A 9-month-old girl sat unaided at 8 months and is now pulling to stand and cruising around furniture. She is not taking any steps on her own but crawls on all fours. She reaches out for objects, which she grasps with a mature palmar grasp and transfers from hand to hand. She uses a pincer grip to pick up a sultana. She babbles constantly but has no clear words.

45. A 6-month-old boy has head lag when pulled to sit, and when held sitting has curved spine and little head control. When placed prone, he lifts his head (but not his chest) briefly and does not attempt to roll over or crawl. He does not reach out for objects, although he fixes and follows them with his eyes. He cries when hungry and makes occasional 'ooh' sounds. He smiles, but not in response to his parents' smiles.

EMQ 10.2 Causes of developmental delay 1

A. Cerebral palsy
B. Chronic illness
C. Deafness
D. Down syndrome
E. Fragile X
F. Hypothyroidism
G. Neglect
H. Phenylketonuria (PKU)
I. Prematurity
J. Tuberous sclerosis

For each of these children, select the most likely cause of their developmental delay:

46. A 2-year-old girl who is the first of triplets attends a hospital clinic for review of previous laser treatment. She wears glasses, and from above her head appears long and narrow from front to back.

47. A 3-year-old boy particularly enjoys the music and singing at his nursery, and is an affectionate child. On examination, he has a sternotomy scar that is well healed, the back of his head is rather flat, and he is small for his age. He is hypotonic and has an unusual face.

48. A 12-month-old girl's parents are taking legal action because a routine blood spot sample was mislaid by the laboratory, and so her condition was not diagnosed until late. She takes a normal diet and is on a single medication, which she takes daily. She has a global delay.

49. A baby girl is admitted acutely at 8 months of age with irritability and fever and is treated for 7 days with intravenous cefotaxime. Several family members receive rifampicin. She makes a good recovery. Two months later, she has a test that was arranged at the time of discharge. Her parents are disappointed but not surprised that it is abnormal.

Learning problems (Chapter 11)

EMQ 11.1   Conditions associated with developmental delay

A. Cerebral palsy
B. Congenital viral infection
C. Down syndrome
D. Emotional neglect
E. Fragile X syndrome
F. Hypothyroidism
G. Idiopathic global developmental delay
H. Tuberous sclerosis

For each of the children, choose the most likely condition:

50. Mark is 9 years old. His teacher notes his difficulty learning to express himself and with reading. He has a number of learning problems. His face is unusual with a prominent jaw and big forehead. His motor function is good.

51. Gary is 8 years old. At 4 months of age, he had infantile spasms. He now has complex partial seizures. He has moderately severe learning problems. On examination, he has a number of pale elliptic patches of skin on his trunk and limbs. He has abnormal fingernails.

52. Sophie is just 6 h old. She has been well since delivery, but she is very floppy and her mother thinks her face looks unusual. She has short fingers and single palmar creases.

53. Susie is 2 years old. She sat unaided at 13 months and walked at 22 months. She walks on tiptoe with her knees and hips flexed. Tone and reflexes in her lower limbs are increased. Otherwise, her development and neurology are normal.

Nutrition (Chapter 13)

EMQ 13.1   Management of nutritional problems

A. Admit to hospital and observe weight gain
B. Give an iron supplement, check diet and follow-up
C. High-energy, high-fat diet with a variety of other foods
D. Reassure and explain that there is nothing to worry about
E. Reduce energy intake by cutting down on fatty and high-energy foods while eating a wide variety of foods

For each of the following, choose the most appropriate management:

54. A baby born at term weighed 2.8 kg (second centile) but appeared well. At 9 months, he remains on the second centile for weight and 2nd–10th centile for length. His parents are convinced that he is well. His development is normal.

55. Jason is 2 years old. He presented with chest infections, diarrhoea and offensive stools. A sweat test is abnormal, and he is homozygous for DF508. His chest is now better, but his weight is on the second centile, height 10th–25th centile.

56. At 17 months of age, Anjali is pale but growing normally along the 50th–75th centile. Haemoglobin is 10.2 g/dL (reference >11 g/dL) with a hypochromic microcytic picture.

EMQ 13.2   Nutritional advice

A. Add thickeners to the milk
B. Advise against breastfeeding
C. Advise that breastfeeding is the best option
D. Prescribe a cow's milk-free formula
E. Stop milk and give glucose electrolyte solution (e.g. Dioralyte)

For each of the following, choose the most appropriate advice:

57. Mrs Phillips has her second child. The first was bottle-fed and has cow's milk allergy with some eczema.

58. Ms Johnson is soon to deliver. She is receiving treatment for HIV.

59. Mrs Passoudi is breastfeeding her 2-month-old son, adding one feed of artificial formula each day. He has diarrhoea but is well.

174. F. This is the normal physiological fall in haemoglobin that occurs over the first 2 months or so in all babies (Chapter 8).

175. G. He has dactylitis. Repeated splenic infarctions may in future years render him asplenic.

EMQ 26.2 Bruising (*see Chapter 26*)

176. F.

177. G. The pattern of injury does not fit the history. A single bruise would be expected (Section 16.2 and Section 16.2.1).

178. D.

EMQ 28.1 Problems of glucose metabolism (*see Chapter 28*)

179. E. This used to be rare in children. It remains unusual and usually occurs in children with obesity.

180. C. Note the normal blood glucose and effect of fasting. Susan's renal threshold is low and she has glycosuria at normal blood glucose levels. No action is needed once diabetes has been excluded.

181. B. This is a rare inborn error of metabolism.

182. D. Classic presentation demanding immediate action to prevent John progressing to diabetic ketoacidosis.

SBA Answers

Chapter 6:

A6.1: d. Cystic fibrosis is an autosomal recessive condition, which is the most common lethal inherited condition amongst Europeans (see Section 20.8 for more details).

A6.2: d. This is a patient with Turner's syndrome, and the most appropriate initial genetic investigation is to identify the characteristic 45XO karyotype. Deletions or mosaicism involving the X chromosome are other possibilities (see Section 14.2.3).

Chapter 7:

A7.1: e. A raised alpha fetoprotein is associated with Spina Bifida, but can also occur in cases of gastroschisis and oesophageal atresia. Chromosomal abnormalities such as Down syndrome are associated with a low alpha fetoprotein level.

A7.2: b. This is a case of Foetal Alcohol Syndrome. These neonates have characteristic facial features as described and intrauterine growth retardation. They may also be irritable and go on to have developmental delay.

Chapter 8:

A8.1: d. In most infants, opening the airway and effective ventilation is all that is required for resuscitation. In this case, initial breaths can be delivered by bag and mask or with a 'T-piece' and mask that allows longer breaths at a set pressure.

A8.2: d. This is a case of posterior urethral valves. Usually, an early ultrasound of the renal tract will be carried out initially. This may show structural changes such as upper tract dilatation. An MCUG would then be performed to confirm the diagnosis (see Section 23.5.6.4 for more details about this investigation)

Chapter 9:

A9.1: d. Jaundice in the first 24 hours is abnormal. The most important causes to consider are haemolysis and sepsis.

A9.2: a. Neonatal sepsis is commonly caused by Group B Streptococcus and *E. Coli.* Benzylpenicillin and Gentamicin are the most appropriate antibiotics in this

Chapter 10:

A10.1: a. This is a case of gross motor delay due to Duchenne muscular dystrophy (DMD). Gower's sign is being described here. This is an X-linked recessive disorder due to a mutation in the dystrophin gene. Creatinine kinase is the most useful initial investigation and this will be markedly elevated in DMD. Genetic analysis looking for abnormalities in the DMD gene is then useful in establishing the diagnosis.

A10.2: c. The combination of findings is consistent with a baby that has been injured by shaking. Injuries in a non-mobile child are concerning and would need a consistent explanation. Knowing appropriate developmental milestones can help with deciding if a mechanism of injury is consistent with the developmental age. Infants usually start rolling at the age of 3–4 months.

Chapter 11:

A11.1: b. Echocardiogram. 50% of children with Down syndrome have a congenital heart defect (mostly atrioventricular septal defect). There is a long-term increased risk of infection, leukaemia, thyroid disorders and diabetes, but those tests are not relevant now.

A11.2: a. A new-onset squint in a young child may indicate a space-occupying lesion (e.g. due to a brain tumour), and he needs urgent imaging. Head tilt is a presenting feature of a brain tumour in a young child (see Section 27.3).

A11.3: b. The description is typical of Fragile X, which probably also affects his younger brother. His mother will be a carrier (but affected less severely). It is due to a triplet repeat on the X chromosome (Section 11.3.2).

Paediatrics Lecture Notes, Tenth Edition. Jonathan C. Darling and James Yong.
© 2022 John Wiley & Sons Ltd. Published 2022 by John Wiley & Sons Ltd.
Companion website: www.wiley.com/go/lecturenotes/paediatrics10e